中医药是中华文化的瑰宝，
是包括汉族和少数民族医药在内的
我国各民族医药的统称。
古人在生命缘起、人体健康、养生寿老、
防病治病、疾病康复等不同阶段，
具有独特的理论认知体系和疾病治疗体系。
因其历史悠久，使用广泛，
为中华人民健康做出了巨大贡献。

Traditional Chinese medicine (TCM) is the treasure of Chinese culture, and it is the general name of all ethnic medicines in China, including Han nationality and ethnic minority medicines. The ancients had unique theoretical cognitive system and disease treatment system in different stages, such as life origin, human health, health preservation and living a long life, preventing and treating diseases, and recovery from diseases. Because of its long history and wide use, it has made significant contributions to the health of the Chinese people.

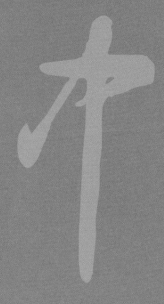

中 医
智 慧 与 健 康 丛书
TCM
Wisdom and Health
Series

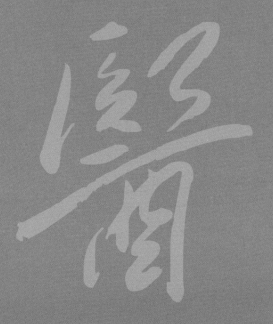

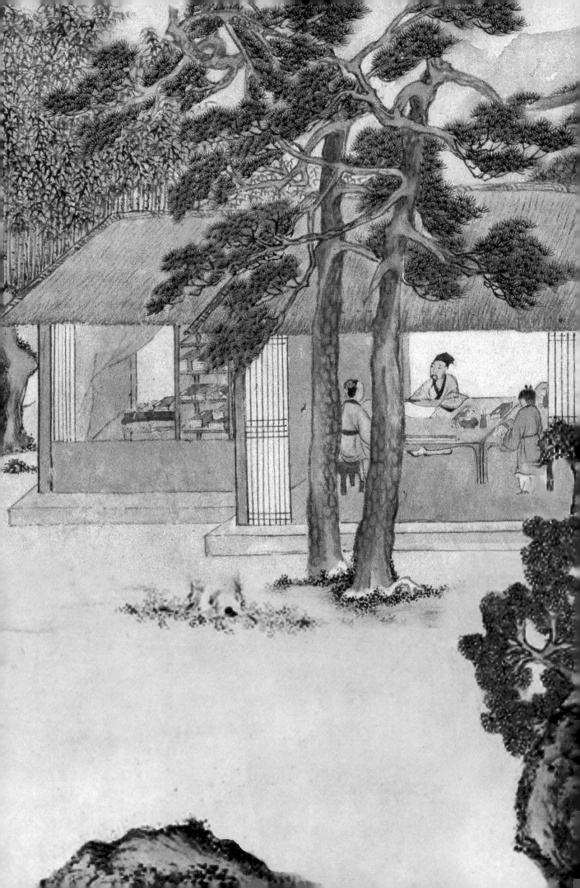

中医诊疗

（汉英对照）

TCM Clinical Diagnosis and Treatment

主　编　王笑频　熊兴江　尹　璐

副主编　王朋倩

编　委（按姓氏笔画排序）

于　悦　王朋倩　王笑频　尹　璐

罗富锟　金子轩　熊兴江

Chief Editors
Wang Xiaopin　Xiong Xingjiang　Yin Lu

Associate Editor
Wang Pengqian

Editorial Board
(Listed in order of surname stroke)

Yu Yue　　　　Wang Pengqian　　Wang Xiaopin　　Yin Lu
Luo Fukun　　Jin Zixuan　　　　Xiong Xingjiang

人民卫生出版社
PMPH　PEOPLE'S MEDICAL PUBLISHING HOUSE

图书在版编目（CIP）数据

中医诊疗：汉英对照 / 王笑频，熊兴江，尹璐主编
. —北京：人民卫生出版社，2023.9
（中医智慧与健康丛书）
ISBN 978-7-117-35057-0

I. ①中… Ⅱ. ①王…②熊…③尹… Ⅲ. ①中医诊
断学－汉、英②中医治疗学－汉、英 Ⅳ. ①R24

中国国家版本馆 CIP 数据核字（2023）第 144661 号

人卫智网	www.ipmph.com	医学教育、学术、考试、健康，购书智慧智能综合服务平台
人卫官网	www.pmph.com	人卫官方资讯发布平台

中医诊疗（汉英对照）
Zhongyi Zhenliao（Han-Ying Duizhao）

主　　编：王笑频　熊兴江　尹　璐
出版发行：人民卫生出版社（中继线 010-59780011）
地　　址：北京市朝阳区潘家园南里 19 号
邮　　编：100021
E - mail：pmph @ pmph.com
购书热线：010-59787592　010-59787584　010-65264830
印　　刷：廊坊一二〇六印刷厂
经　　销：新华书店
开　　本：710×1000　1/16　印张：15
字　　数：294 千字
版　　次：2023 年 9 月第 1 版
印　　次：2023 年 9 月第 1 次印刷
标准书号：ISBN 978-7-117-35057-0
定　　价：128.00 元

打击盗版举报电话：010-59787491　E-mail：WQ @ pmph.com
质量问题联系电话：010-59787234　E-mail：zhiliang @ pmph.com
数字融合服务电话：4001118166　　E-mail：zengzhi @ pmph.com

序

　　中医药蕴含着数千年来中华民族治病疗疾、养生保健的智慧，护佑着中华儿女生生不息，是中华民族的伟大创造与中国古代科学的瑰宝。《中医智慧与健康丛书》正是为了系统总结中医药千年来的实践经验与临床智慧、科学普及中医药知识所编撰。

　　本丛书由中国中医科学院广安门医院牵头撰写，依托国家中医药管理局国际合作司中医药国际合作专项，通过《中医史话》《中华本草》《中医诊疗》《中医养生》四个分册，全方位展示了中医药历史传承、特色优势和优秀成果，旨在向国内外读者普及中医药文化，促进中医药文化的国际传播，做好文明互鉴。丛书精心选取内容，语言通俗易懂，图文并茂，采用中英双语对照的形式，以方便国内外读者阅读。

　　我们真诚地希望通过本丛书，广大读者朋友能够更好地了解中医、用上中医、爱上中医，成为中医的"粉丝"。

《中医智慧与健康丛书》编委会
2023 年 6 月

TCM Wisdom
and
Health Series

Foreword

Traditional Chinese medicine (TCM) contains the wisdom of the Chinese nation in treating diseases and maintaining health for thousands of years, and protects the endless survival of the Chinese people. It is the great creation of the Chinese nation and the treasure of ancient Chinese science. The *TCM Wisdom and Health Series* is compiled to systematically summarize the practical experience and clinical wisdom of TCM and popularize the knowledge of TCM.

This series is compiled under the leadership of Guang'anmen Hospital of China Academy of Chinese Medical Sciences (CACMS). Relying on the Special International Cooperation Project of TCM of Department of International Cooperation of National Administration of Traditional Chinese Medicine, the series shows the historical inheritance, characteristic advantages and outstanding achievements of TCM in an all-round way ranging from history, materia medica, diagnosis and treatment of TCM to health cultivation, aiming to popularize Chinese medical culture to readers at home and abroad, promote the international communication of Chinese medical culture as well as mutual learning among civilizations. The series carefully selects content, uses language easy to understand, illustrates texts with pictures, and adopts the bilingual form of both Chinese and English to facilitate readers at home and abroad.

We sincerely hope by reading this series readers can better understand TCM, use TCM, fall in love with TCM, and become the "fans" of TCM.

Editorial Board of ***TCM Wisdom and Health Series***

June 2023

前 言

中医药是中华文化的瑰宝，是包括汉族和少数民族医药在内的我国各民族医药的统称。古人在生命缘起、人体健康、养生寿老、防病治病、疾病康复等不同阶段，具有独特的理论认知体系和疾病治疗体系。因其历史悠久，使用广泛，为中华人民健康做出了巨大贡献。

在理论认识上，中医学对人体生命活动和疾病变化规律的理论包括阴阳、五行、八纲、脏象、经络、病因、病机、诊法、辨证、治法、预防、养生等内容。

在临床诊疗上，中医学对疾病的分科虽然没有特别详细，但大致也可以分为中医内科、中医外科、中医妇科、中医儿科、中医眼科等。《金匮要略》《中藏经》《外科正宗》《济阴纲目》《小儿药证直诀》《秘传眼科龙木论》等都是古代医家的临床分科代表作。《史记·扁鹊仓公列传》也记载了当时疾病分科的朴素理念，"扁鹊名闻天下，过邯郸，闻贵妇人，即为带下医；过雒阳，闻周人爱老人，即为耳目痹医；来入咸阳，闻秦人爱小儿，即为小儿医，随俗为变。"

在诊疗方法上，中医药学中既有药物疗法，包括中药、经典名方，以及现代常用的中成药剂型，又包括针刺、太极、八段锦、五禽戏、气功、艾灸、拔罐、刮痧在内的非药物疗法。

近年来，青蒿素治疗疟疾，三氧化二砷治疗白血病，太极拳治疗高血压，麻仁丸治疗便秘，针刺治疗压力性尿失禁等逐渐受到国际主流医学和权威杂志的认可。我们将在本书中，以图文并茂的方式和通俗易懂的语言介绍常见疾病的中医认识及治疗手段，展示中医药的疗效证据。希望本书的出版能够为科普中医药的临床治疗理念，推进中医药的国际化进程，贡献出一份力量。

限于编写水平，本书难免有不尽如人意之处，望各位读者对本书的缺点和错误及时指正，以便我们勘误或再版时更正，敬请各位不吝赐教。

《中医诊疗》编写委员会
2023 年 6 月

Preface

Traditional Chinese medicine (TCM) is the treasure of Chinese culture, and it is the general name of all ethnic medicines in China, including Han nationality and ethnic minority medicines. The ancients had unique theoretical cognitive system and disease treatment system in different stages, such as life origin, human health, health preservation and living a long life, preventing and treating diseases, and recovery from diseases. Because of its long history and wide use, it has made significant contributions to the health of the Chinese people.

The theories of TCM on human life activities and disease changes include yin and yang, five elements, eight principles, visceral manifestations, meridians, etiology, pathogenesis, diagnostic method, syndrome differentiation, method of treatment, prevention, health preservation, and so on.

In clinical diagnosis and treatment, although the classification of diseases in TCM is not particularly detailed, it can be roughly divided into internal medicine of TCM, surgery of TCM, gynecology of TCM, pediatrics of TCM, ophthalmology of TCM, and so on. *Synopsis of Golden Chamber*, *The Treasured Classics*, *Orthodox Manual of External Diseases*, *Outline for Women's Diseases*, *Key to Therapeutics of Children's Diseases*, and *Nagarjuna's Ophthalmology Secretly Handed Down* are all representative works of disease classification of ancient doctors. *Historical Records–Bianque Canggong Liezhuan* also recorded the simple concept of disease classification at that time:"Bianque is famous all over the world. When he arrived in Handan, he heard that the people of the State of Zhao respected women, so he became a gynecologist. When he arrived in Luoyang, he heard that the people of the Zhou Dynasty respected the elderly, so he became a geriatrician.

When he arrived in Xianyang, he heard that the people of Qin loved their children, so he became a pediatrician. He always changed the emphasis of his practice of medicine as customs changed."

In terms of diagnosis and treatment methods, there are not only medicine therapies, including Chinese medicinals, classic prescriptions, and modern commonly used dosage forms of Chinese patent medicine, but also non-medicine therapies, including acupuncture, Tai Chi, Baduanjin, Wuqinxi, Qigong, moxibustion, cupping, and scraping.

In recent years, artemisinin for malaria, arsenic trioxide for leukemia, Tai Chi for hypertension, Maren Pill for constipation, and acupuncture for stress urinary incontinence have been gradually recognized by international mainstream medicine and authoritative journals. Therefore, in the book, we focus on how TCM understands and treats the most common diseases. Through the forms of illustrations and plain language, the evidence of the efficacy of TCM is shown. The publication of this book is expected to contribute to popularizing the clinical treatment concept of TCM and promoting the internationalization of TCM by summarizing the latest curative effect evidence.

Due to limitation of knowledge, there will inevitably be some unsatisfactory points. We hope readers can correct the shortcomings and mistakes of this book in time, so we can revise them when we make errata or reprint them. Please give us your advice.

Editorial Board of
TCM Clinical Diagnosis and Treatment
June 2023

目 录

Contents

目　录

Contents

Contents

Contents

中医诊疗
（汉英对照）

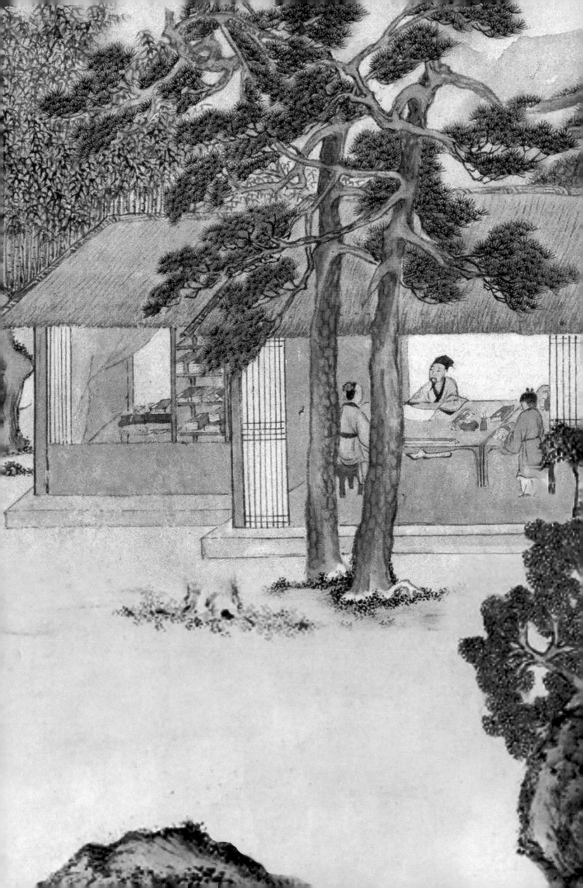

第一章

中医药疗法简介

第一节
药物疗法

一、中药

中药是指在中国传统医药理论指导下，通过对药材的采集、炮制、制剂，用于预防、治疗、诊断疾病，具有康复与保健作用，并能够指导中医药临床应用的药物。中药主要来源于天然药及其加工品，包括植物药、动物药、矿物药及部分化学、生物制品类药物。"诸药以草为本"，在这5个亚类中，中药尤其以植物药多见。

在这里，重点介绍单味药、有效成分及膳食补充剂的临床运用。单味中药治病在古代早有记载，属于中药配伍七情中的"单行"。在《神农本草经·序录》中，将各种药物的配伍关系归纳为"有单行者，有相须者，有相使者，有相畏者，有相恶者，有相反者，有相杀者，凡此七情，合和视之"。《本草纲目·序例》中也说"独行者，单方不用辅也"。单行，就是临床单独运用一味中药来治疗某种病情单一的病症。面对病情比较单纯的疾病，选择一种针对性较强的药物即可达到治疗目的。在《伤寒论》中，共有4首处方运用单味药治病，包括《伤寒论》太阳病篇第141条文蛤散（文蛤）、阳明病篇第233条蜜煎导方（蜜）、少阴病篇第311条甘草汤（甘草）、阴阳易差后劳复病篇第392条烧裈散。在古代，独参汤就是单用一味中药人参，治疗大失血之后导致的元气虚脱的危重症；清金散就是单用一味中药黄芩，治疗肺热导致咳血的病症。其他还包括：《神农本草经》中记载一味黄连治疗下利；一味马齿苋治疗痢疾；一味夏枯草膏消瘿瘤；一味益母草膏活血调经，通络止痛；一味鹤草根芽驱杀绦虫等，都是临床治病的有效方法。

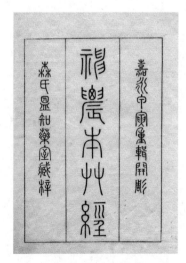

《神农本草经》

中药有效成分是指来源于中药的化学上的单体化合物，对生物体代谢或者化学反应起作用的成分，并且在中药材中起主要药效作用。有效成分一般能用分子式和结构式表示，如麻黄碱、青蒿素等。这种致力于从天然药物中筛选化学新药的研究思路，在近几十年来的研究历程中取得显著成就。例如，治疗疟疾的青蒿素，抗肿瘤的紫杉醇，解痉平喘的左旋麻黄素，活血化瘀、通络止痛的丹参酚酸盐，活血通络的丹参酮 II_A 磺酸钠等。

膳食补充剂是指来自于天然药物，或通过化学或生物技术生产而成的，包括动植物提取物、维生素、矿物质、氨基酸、膳食纤维等。在美国，膳食补充剂源于美国食品药品监督管理局 1994 年颁布的《膳食补充剂健康与教育法》（DSHEA），被称为"dietary supplement"。膳食补充剂一般以片剂或胶囊剂为主要剂型。通过口服膳食补充剂，补充人体所必需的营养素和生物活性物质，达到促进机体健康，减少疾病发作的目标。一般而言，膳食补充剂中所含有活性物质成分结构明确，理化性质稳定，作用机制清晰。膳食补充剂在现今临床运用尤其普遍。大量的中药被归属于膳食补充剂范畴，包括大蒜素、红曲、银杏叶制剂等。

二、经典名方

经典名方是指在中医药理论指导下，历经千百年临床锤炼而成的中医方剂。因其源自于古代经典医籍或有代表性的古代中医著作，临床疗效确切，为历代中医学家广泛运用，并且一直沿用至今。在现今临床中，经典名方一直广泛运用于临床各科的疾病治疗。包括麻杏石甘汤治疗肺炎，天麻钩藤饮治疗高血压，炙甘草汤治疗心肌炎，半夏泻心汤治疗慢性胃炎，小柴胡汤治疗感染性发热，镇肝熄风汤治疗急性脑梗死等。

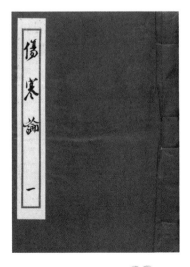

《伤寒论》

中国中医科学院馆藏

三、中成药

中成药是指将中药材按照一定的原则加工而制成各种不同剂型的中药制品，包括丸、散、膏、丹等各种剂型。中成药运用历史悠久，是我国历代中医学家经过数千年临床实践总结而成的有效方剂的精华。中成药可以分为内服和外用两种。内服中成药的常用剂型包括丸剂、散剂、颗粒剂、片剂、胶囊剂等，可运用于脏腑气血功能失调所导致的各种疾病。外用中成药常用的剂型包括膏贴剂、酊剂、搽剂、栓剂、滴鼻剂、滴眼剂、气雾剂等，可运用于外科、外伤、皮肤科、五官科等多种疾病。中成药因其组成固定，适用面广，能够广泛用于临床各科疾病，其不足则在于不可随意加减。

按照药物的临床功效，中成药可以分为解表类、泻下类、清热类、温里类、补益类、安神类、固涩类、理气类、理血类、祛湿类、治风类、祛痰类、止咳平喘类、消导类等。在临床中，中成药临床运用极为普遍，例如速效救心丸治疗冠心病心绞痛，脑立清丸治疗脑梗死头晕头痛，藿香正气软胶囊治疗急慢性胃肠炎、胃肠型感冒，逍遥颗粒治疗女性胸胁胀痛、月经不调，桂枝茯苓丸治疗妇科子宫肌瘤，活血止痛膏治疗关节痛等。

第二节
非药物疗法

一、针刺

针刺疗法是指在中医学理论指导下，将针具（通常指毫针）按照一定的角度刺入患者体内，综合运用捻转、提插等针刺手法来对人体特定部位（穴位）进行刺激，具有通经活络、活血化瘀等功效，从而达到治疗疾病目的。刺入点称为人体腧穴，简称穴位。

根据不同针刺用具的形制、用途、刺激方式，针刺疗法可以分为毫针疗法、皮肤针疗法、皮内针疗法、火针疗法、水针疗法、鍉针疗法、电针疗法、刺络疗法、圆利针疗法等。针刺疗法具有适应证广泛，疗效显著，操作简单、方便，安全经济等优点，深受广大临床医生和患者的欢迎。

以心血管疾病为例，作为中医药中应用最广泛的非药物疗法，针刺不仅可改善冠心病、高血压、心律失常等患者胸闷、头晕、头痛、心慌等临床不适症状，而且能减少发作频次，平稳降压，减少并发症及靶器官损害，具有一定的临床价值与意义。

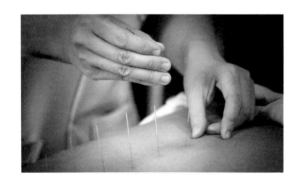

针刺操作

二、太极拳

太极拳是一种传统武术项目，也是体育运动和健身项目，在中国有着悠久的历史。太极拳是根据古代《易经》阴阳原理，中医经络学说，道家导引、吐纳，综合创造的一套有阴阳性质，符合人体结构、自然规律的一种拳术。太极拳融合了我国传统阴阳五行理论，通过动与静相互结合转化，促进脏腑的气血循环，改善脏腑功能，使身心处于和谐平衡。在现代临床中，太极拳也被广泛用于各种慢性疾病的治疗与康复，包括慢性阻塞性肺疾病、高血压、冠心病、脑梗死、帕金森病等疾病。

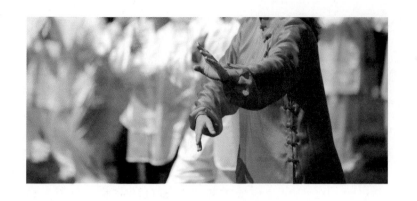

三、八段锦

八段锦起源于北宋时期，至今已经有八百多年历史。根据北宋洪迈《夷坚志》中的描述，"政和七年，李似矩为起居郎……嘘吸按摩，行所谓八段锦者"。八段锦一共有八个动作，包括两手托天理三焦，左右开弓似射雕，调理脾胃须单举，五劳七伤往后瞧，摇头摆尾去心火，两手攀足固肾腰，攒拳怒目增气力，背后七颠百病消。古代把这套动作比喻为"锦"，即有五颜六色、美丽华贵之意。

与剧烈运动相比，八段锦对体力要求更低。八段锦因动作简单、舒缓而广泛应用于多种疾病的治疗，包括高血压、糖尿病、高脂血症、高尿酸血症、睡眠障碍、颈椎病、腰椎疾病、焦虑、抑郁状态等。中国健身气功协会建议在社区推广八段锦，改善高血压患者血压水平、临床症状及生活质量，这有益于提高心脏病患者的活动耐量。

四、五禽戏

五禽戏是中国传统导引养生的一个重要功法，由三国时期的医家华佗（约145—208）创制而成。五禽戏效仿五种动物，即虎、鹿、熊、猿、鸟（鹤）的活动，而进行的健身运动，对躯体及五脏都有良好的锻炼效果，所传颇广。据《后汉书·方术列传·华佗传》记载："吾有一术，名五禽之戏：一曰虎，二曰鹿，三曰熊，四曰猿，五曰鸟。亦以除疾，兼利蹄足，以当导引。体有不快，起作一禽之戏，怡而汗出，因以著粉，身体轻便而欲食。普施行之，年九十余，耳目聪明，齿牙完坚。"华佗弟子中，著名者有吴普、樊阿、李当之等人。其中，吴普著有《吴普本草》，据传他练习五禽戏，活到100多岁。现代也将五禽戏广泛用于内分泌代谢性疾病、骨关节疾病等慢性疾病。

五、气功

气功也是一种中国传统保健、养生、祛病方法。气功是以调整呼吸，身体活动和意识（调息、调身、调心）为手段，通过韵律动作、呼吸吐纳，配合心理冥想，调节经络以及脏腑器官功能，促进气血运行，达到强身健体、防病治病、延年益寿等目的的一种身心锻炼方法。现在已经将气功广泛用于高血压、冠心病、失眠、脑梗死、骨关节疾病等慢性疾病。

六、艾灸

灸法，古称"灸焫""艾灸"，是以灸炷或灸草在体表特定的经络腧穴进行烧灼、熏熨，借助火的温热给穴位以温性刺激，具有温经散寒、扶阳固脱、消瘀散结等功效，有预防和治疗疾病的作用。临床以艾草最为常用，故又称为艾灸。另有隔药灸、柳条灸、灯心灸、桑枝灸等方法。现今，临床使用最多的是艾条灸。

艾灸在临床被广泛运用于骨关节疾病的寒性疼痛，包括膝关节疼痛、膝骨性关节炎、颈椎病、腰椎病、肩周炎等。艾灸还可用于部分内科疾病，包括慢性腹泻、慢性寒性腹痛、寒性痛经等。另外，艾灸还有一定的温补阳气作用，可用于阳虚体质的调理。

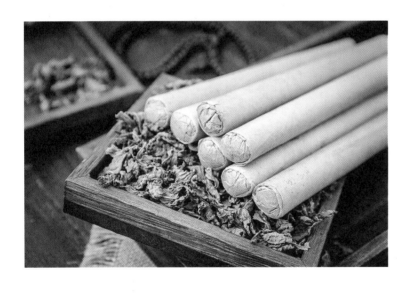

艾条

七、拔罐

拔罐以罐为工具，主要利用燃火和抽气等方法排空罐内空气，形成负压，使罐吸附于相应腧穴及特定部位的体表，使局部皮肤充血、瘀血，达到通经活络、行气活血、消肿止痛、祛风散寒目的。拔罐疗法有着悠久历史。早在《五十二病方》中就有关于"角法"（类似于后世的火罐疗法）的记载。拔罐可分为火罐法、水罐法、抽吸罐法等。现今临床上，拔罐疗法被广泛用于治疗风湿痹痛、肩背疼痛、哮喘、胃痛、腹痛、腹泻、痛经、痤疮、荨麻疹、面瘫等疾病。

八、刮痧

刮痧是传统的中医疗法之一，是以中医皮部理论为基础，用牛角、玉石、火罐等器具在皮肤相关部位刮拭，以达到疏通经络、活血化瘀的目的。刮痧可用于治疗颈椎病、感寒、中暑、受风、肠胃病、肩背痛、皮肤病等。

九、推拿

推拿也是一种中医传统疗法，是指在人体的经络、穴位，综合运用推、拿、提、捏、揉等手法进行治疗，以期达到疏通经络、调和气血、通络止痛、祛邪扶正、调和阴阳、延年益寿的目的。其起源可追溯到上古时期，又称为摩挲、按跷、按摩。在《素问·异法方宜论》中明确指出："中央者，其地平以湿，天地所以生万物也众，其民食杂而不劳，故其病多痿厥寒热，其治宜导引按跷，故导引按跷者，亦从中央出也。"在《素问·血气形志》中也指出："形乐志苦，病生于脉，治之以灸刺。形乐志乐，病生于肉，治之以针石。形苦志乐，病生于筋，治之以熨引。形苦志苦，病生于咽嗌，治之以百药。形数惊恐，经络不通，病生于不仁，治之以按摩醪药。"

现今临床中，推拿常用于治疗筋骨病，包括腰椎间盘突出症、肩周炎、腰痛、颈椎病。另外，部分儿科类疾病，如食积、腹痛、腹泻、发热、咳嗽等，也可采用推拿疗法。

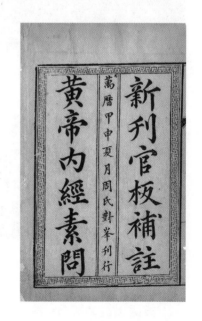

《黄帝内经素问》

第二章

常见疾病的

中医诊疗智慧

第一节
呼吸系统疾病

一、呼吸系统疾病概述

咳嗽、咳痰、气喘……相信大家都有过类似的经历，一般医生都会告知这是"肺不好""感冒了"……实际上，这些都是呼吸系统疾病的常见症状。呼吸系统疾病作为一种常见病、多发病，主要病变部位在气管、支气管、肺部及胸腔，轻者表现为咳嗽、咳痰、胸痛、呼吸费力，严重的会导致呼吸困难、缺氧，甚至死亡。常见呼吸系统疾病包括急性上呼吸道感染、肺炎、慢性阻塞性肺疾病、支气管哮喘、肺部结节等。

在临床治疗上，治疗药物包括抗生素、支气管扩张剂、痰液稀释剂、抗过敏药物等。然而，我们发现，仍有很多儿童因抵抗力差反复出现上呼吸道感染；老年患者对抗生素不敏感，治疗肺炎疗效不佳；慢性阻塞性肺疾病受凉后就反复发作；支气管哮喘的孩子必须随身携带噻托溴铵、沙美特罗替卡松等解痉药；肺部结节患者在结节小于 1 cm 时只能定期复查而无任何手段干预……

近年来，中医药治疗呼吸系统疾病的临床价值越来越受到国际认可。尤其是在新型冠状病毒感染的防治中，中医药在退热、缩短发热病程上的疗效得到重视与认可。其实中医学对呼吸系统疾病具有独特的认知体系和治疗方药。呼吸系统疾病属于中医"咳嗽""感冒""哮病""喘证""肺胀"等疾病范畴，其病位主要在肺，主要病机为肺失宣降，肺气不利，并与全身各个脏腑密切相关。研究发现，中医药在快速退热，缓解咳嗽、咳痰症状，减少慢性阻塞性肺疾病和支气管哮喘的发作频次，改善生活质量等方面显示出一定价值。本节将重点讨论中医药对急性上呼吸道感染、支气管哮喘、肺部结节、慢性阻塞性肺疾病、甲型流行性感冒的认识与治疗。

二、呼吸系统疾病各论

1. 急性上呼吸道感染

急性上呼吸道感染，俗称感冒，是包括鼻腔、咽或喉部急性炎症的总称。在临床症状上，本病常见的临床表现包括喷嚏、鼻塞、流涕、咳嗽、咳痰、咽部不适、流泪、发热、恶寒、乏力、头痛、呼吸不畅、声嘶、颌下淋巴结肿大疼痛等。

在临床诊断上，除了不适症状外，还需结合发病经过、血常规、细菌病毒培养结果，才能明确诊断及指导合理用药。

在临床治疗上，除对症治疗外，使用频率最高、最为老百姓所知晓的就是抗生素，也就是俗称的"消炎药"。对一部分人群来说，应用抗生素的确能够药到病除，但前提是在合适的时机，选择合适的剂量和种类。遗憾的是，抗生素大量长期使用易产生耐药及相关不良反应，包括肠道菌群失调、抗生素相关腹泻等，在一定程度上影响了临床疗效。

其实，在本病初期，很多患者会选择服用中药。如果治疗及时，能够迅速阻断疾病进展而愈。中医学认为，急性上呼吸道感染属于"感冒"范畴，其病因主要以外感为主，或兼有正气不足。

在临床治疗上，常用小柴胡颗粒和感冒清热颗粒。经典名方小柴胡汤出自《伤寒论》，由柴胡、黄芩、半夏、生姜、人参、大枣、甘草7味中药组成，具有和解少阳的功效。在古代，小柴胡汤主要用于治疗伤寒少阳证。在上呼吸道感染的患者中，如果发热的同时伴有呕吐，或者出现口苦，口干，咽痛，食欲不振，这就是我们用小柴胡颗粒的典型适应证。值得注意的是，在北方，很多人受凉了之后立刻会"上嗓子"，马上会说嗓子不舒服，患者都会说这是上火了，其实这就是中医说的小柴胡汤/颗粒的指征。小柴胡颗粒用法用量：开水冲服，每次1~2袋，每天3次。

感冒清热颗粒是后世医家研制的处方，由荆芥穗、薄荷、防风、柴胡、紫苏叶、葛根、桔梗、苦杏仁、白芷、苦地丁、芦根11味中药组成，具有疏风散寒、解表清热的功效。本方可用于治疗风寒兼有郁而化热的感冒。与小柴胡颗粒主治口苦、咽干、咽痛不同的是，当患者既出现头痛发热、恶寒身痛、鼻流清涕、咳嗽等表寒症状，又出现咽干、小便黄等内热症状，就可以用感冒清热颗粒。感冒清热颗粒用法用量：开水冲服，每次1袋，每天2次。

2. 支气管哮喘

日常生活中我们经常会见到一些人，他们无论走到哪儿，口袋里总会装着一瓶喷嗓子的药，而这些人所患的就是俗称的"哮喘病"。

这种"哮喘病"的学名为支气管哮喘，是由嗜酸性粒细胞、肥大细胞等多种细胞参与的气道慢性炎症性疾病。它的典型症状为发作性呼吸困难，以呼气相为主，甚至强迫坐位，常伴有哮鸣音，或伴有咳嗽、咳痰、胸闷、面部及口唇青紫等。部分患者仅表现为咳嗽，这种类型称为咳嗽变异性哮喘；有的患者，尤其是青少年，其发病总是在运动时出现胸闷、咳嗽及呼吸困难，这一类型称为运动性哮喘。

在发病诱因上，包括尘螨、花粉、吸入冷空气、药物及某些食物。本病可在数分钟内发作，持续时间在数小时至数天不等。

在临床诊断上，除了典型的呼吸困难、哮鸣音等临床症状外，还需结合发病经过，以及血常规、过敏原测定、胸片、肺功能测定、血气分析等专科检查结果才能确诊。

在临床治疗上，人们最熟知的药物包括解痉药布地奈德福莫特罗、沙美特罗替卡松等。然而，部分患者在用药后可能会出现血糖升高、骨质疏松、免疫力下降、药物耐受、疗效下降等诸多反应。还有部分患者因支气管哮喘反复发作，用药后即能缓解，停药后复发，深以为苦，进而来门诊寻求中医药治疗。中医药在减轻支气管哮喘发作时的呼吸困难症状、减少发作频次，停减西药上具有一定的临床优势。

在中医学中，支气管哮喘属于"哮病"范畴。在病因上，包括外邪侵袭、饮食不当、体虚、病后、情志变化、劳倦以及家族禀赋。在病机上，本病与宿痰伏肺、正气亏虚有关。

在临床治疗时，需要区分支气管哮喘属于急性加重期，还是缓解期。对正处在急性加重期，短时间内发病频繁、症状严重的，射干麻黄汤是常用的经典名方。射干麻黄汤出自《金匮要略》，由射干、麻黄、生姜、细辛、紫菀、款冬花、五味子、大枣、半夏9味中药组成，能温肺散寒、化痰平喘。本方适用于哮喘伴见呼吸急促，喉中哮鸣有声，胸部憋闷，轻微咳嗽，咳少量白黏痰，口不渴，或渴喜热饮，天冷或遇寒而发，形寒怕冷，或有恶寒，喷嚏，流涕患者。现代临床研究表明，射干麻黄汤能降低气道高反应性。

而在支气管哮喘的缓解期，常用中成药玉屏风颗粒以增强体质、改善肺功能、减少发作频次等。玉屏风颗粒出自《世医得效方》，由黄芪、防风、白术3味中药组成，具有益气、固表、止汗之功效。在支气管哮喘的缓解期，如果见到气短、活动后加重，怕风，整日出汗不断，稍微吹风就容易感冒，或喉中有轻度哮鸣声，咳痰清稀色白时，可以口服玉屏风颗粒来增强体质。用法用量为每次5g，每日3次。

参考文献

LIN C C, WANG Y Y, CHEN S M, et al. Shegan-Mahuang Decoction ameliorates asthmatic airway hyperresponsiveness by downregulating Th2/Th17 cells but upregulating CD4[+] FoxP3+ Tregs[J]. Journal of Ethnopharmacology, 2020, 253: e112656.

3. 肺部结节

许多人平时没有什么不舒服，身体很健康，只是在单位体检拍胸片的时候，查出来肺上长了个结节，就吓得不知所措，以为自己得了不治之症。从医学上讲，肺结节是指肺部影像上各种大小、边缘清楚或模糊、直径小于或等于 3cm 的局灶性圆形致密影。

在发病原因上，肺结节的形成可能与吸烟、空气污染、工业粉尘颗粒吸入、肺部疾病后遗症相关。肺结节的确有恶性的可能，但并不是只要有肺结节就意味着"得病了"，也并不是所有的肺结节都需要治疗。因此，当查出肺部有结节时，先不要慌张，应积极寻求专业医生的帮助，听从医生的建议。

肺结节的良恶性鉴别，除了根据影像学结果，还需要结合患者的临床症状、病史、职业特点、生活习惯，以及血常规、痰液培养、结核杆菌、肿瘤标志物等检验结果，尤其是肺部结节的穿刺结果，经慎重评估，才能最终明确诊断。

在查出患有肺结节的人群中，当其直径小于 1cm，但没有任何不适症状，各项血液检查和痰培养结果都正常，这类患者可以观察 3 个月后再复查。如果结节没有继续增大，可定期复查。若发现结节明显增大，则需穿刺取病理组织进行活检，根据病理结果决定下一步治疗方案。

在临床治疗中，很多患者不愿意被动等待，而寄希望于中医药，通过改善生活方式，结合内服中药软坚散结、化痰活血，以期能在 3 个月后的复查中达到缩小结节的目的。

在中医学中，根据其临床症状，肺部结节可归属于"咳嗽""喘证""肺痨""肺癌"等范畴。在病机上，肺部结节属于有形之邪，多与气滞、痰浊、瘀血内停、阻滞经络有关。根据中医学的临床经验，常用小柴胡汤、消瘰丸，但是目前还缺乏循证证据支持。

小柴胡汤出自《伤寒论》，由柴胡、黄芩、半夏、生姜、人参、大枣、甘草7 味中药组成，具有和解少阳之功效。我们发现，很多肺部结节患者均存在一定的肝气郁结、气滞不通的指征，如伴见胸闷、心烦、食欲减退、恶心、呕吐、口干、口苦、头晕、目眩等。因此可以小柴胡汤为基础方，随症加减。

消瘰丸出自清代医家程钟龄的《医学心悟》，由浙贝母、玄参、牡蛎 3 味中药组成，具有清润化痰、软坚散结之功效。中医学认为肺部结节与痰浊阻滞有关。本方适用于肺部结节伴见咳嗽、咳痰，痰黄质黏稠、胸闷、气促、口渴、喜冷饮，舌红、苔黄等症状的患者。

4. 慢性阻塞性肺疾病

我们时常见到这样的患者，他们看上去胸腔是圆柱形的，好像一个水桶，似乎一直提着一口气一样，稍微走快一点就气喘吁吁，咳个不停。在平时安静状态下，呼吸浅而快，时不时地大口喘气、咳嗽、咳痰。这些人多半是得了"慢性阻塞性肺疾病"。

慢性阻塞性肺疾病，俗称"慢阻肺"，是一种以持续性气流阻塞为特征的慢性支气管炎或肺气肿。慢性支气管炎，俗称"慢支"，是指在排除其他具有咳嗽、咳痰、喘息症状的疾病后，每年咳嗽、咳痰持续3个月以上，连续2年或2年以上者。肺气肿是指肺部终末细支气管远端出现异常持久的扩张，同时存在细支气管和肺泡的破坏而无明显的肺纤维化改变。当慢支和肺气肿患者肺功能检查提示持续性气流受限时，就可以诊断为慢性阻塞性肺疾病了。

在病因上，本病与吸烟、长期接触高浓度职业粉尘、反复呼吸道感染、高龄，以及免疫功能紊乱等诸多因素有关。在临床症状上，包括慢性咳嗽、咳痰、喘息、胸闷。在临床诊断上，除上述症状外，查体时可以见到患者的胸廓前后径增大，呈"桶状胸"，还需要结合病史、生活习惯和环境，辅助检查（胸片、肺 CT 等，尤其是肺功能检查）结果，方可确诊。

在临床治疗上，多采用对症治疗，常用的药物如沙美特罗替卡松、噻托溴铵、硫酸沙丁胺醇、二羟丙茶碱等，可以说是慢性阻塞性肺疾病患者的"老朋友"了。这些药见效迅速、携带方便，在发作时能有效减轻症状。但是，仍然有部分人群使用后会出现胃肠道不适、心慌等副作用，药物过敏，或者因疗效变差而反复发作，生活质量受到影响。

中医药治疗慢性阻塞性肺疾病，能够缓解临床症状、减少发作频率，同时还能增强患者体质。在中医学中，慢性阻塞性肺疾病属于"肺胀"范畴。在病因上，每因感受外邪而发作或加重。在病机上，多与久病肺虚，痰浊潴留，而致肺气胀满，失于敛降有关。主要症状为胸部膨满，憋闷如塞，喘息上气，咳嗽痰多。

在临床治疗上，常用小青龙汤和射干麻黄汤。小青龙汤出自《伤寒论》，由麻黄、桂枝、白芍、甘草、干姜、细辛、半夏、五味子8味中药组成，具有解表散寒、温肺化饮之功效。原文写道："咳逆倚息不得卧，小青龙汤主之""伤寒，心下有水气，咳而微喘，发热不渴"。慢性阻塞性肺疾病患者在受凉后出现剧烈咳嗽、气喘，不能平躺，咳泡沫样稀白痰，怕冷，浑身酸疼，不想喝水或想喝热水等症状，可以选用小青龙汤，水煎服，或中药配方颗粒剂开水冲服，每日1剂，早晚各服药1次。

射干麻黄汤出自《金匮要略》，原文记载其适应证为"咳而上气，喉中水鸡声"。本方由射干、麻黄、生姜、细辛、紫菀、款冬花、五味子、大枣、半夏9味中药组成，具有温肺散寒、化痰平喘之功效。本方适用于慢性阻塞性肺疾病急性加重期，症见呼吸急促，喉中哮鸣有声，胸部憋闷，轻微咳嗽，咳少量白黏痰，口不渴，或渴喜热饮，天冷或遇寒而发，形寒怕冷，或有恶寒，喷嚏，流涕患者。中药饮片水煎服，或中药配方颗粒剂开水冲服，每日1剂，早晚各服药1次。

参考文献

KAO S T, WANG S T, YU C K, et al. The effect of Chinese herbal medicine, xiao-qing-long tang (XQLT), on allergen-induced bronchial inflammation in mite-sensitized mice[J]. Allergy, 2000, 55(12): 1127-1133.

5. 甲型流行性感冒

尽管距离甲型H1N1流行性感冒暴发已经过去10年之久，相信大家仍然对它难以忘怀。甲型流行性感冒，俗称"甲流"，是由甲型流感病毒引起的急性呼吸道传染病。H和N分别是指甲型流感病毒血凝素H和神经氨酸酶N，H有15种，N有9种，所谓的H1N1，即是甲型流感病毒的其中一种亚型。

甲型流行性感冒主要通过接触和空气飞沫传播，北方冬、春季多发，南方全年均可流行。人感染甲流后的早期症状与普通感冒十分相似。不同的是，甲流起病急，有明显的流行性和暴发性，畏寒、高热、头痛、全身肌肉酸痛等中毒症状明显，鼻咽部症状较轻，有些患者还会出现眼结膜炎、腹泻或呕吐、食欲减退等。病情严重者可并发重症肺炎，甚至因休克、呼吸衰竭等而死亡。

在临床诊断上，除发病经过和临床症状外，还需结合血常规，鼻咽部、下呼吸道分泌物或口腔含漱液病原学检查，血清病毒抗原及抗体检测结果，方可明确诊断。

在临床治疗上，对疑似和确诊患者，首先要进行隔离，在常规应用抗病毒药物如奥司他韦、帕拉米韦的基础上，进行对症治疗和支持治疗。除了病毒毒力外，自身免疫状况是决定预后的重要因素。单纯性甲流一般预后较好，而年老体弱患者容易合并肺炎、毒血症等并发症，易进展为重症，且治疗过程中常继发细菌感染。

中医药在快速退热、截断病程发展、增强患者体质、减少重症病例方面都具有显著优势。在中医学中，甲流归属于"时行感冒"范畴。在病因上，为感受时行病毒所诱发。在病机上，多与邪犯肺卫，卫表失和有关。

在临床治疗中，常用银翘散和麻杏石甘汤。银翘散出自清代医家吴鞠通的《温病条辨》，由连翘、金银花、桔梗、薄荷、竹叶、甘草、荆芥、淡豆豉、牛蒡子、芦根 10 味中药组成，具有辛凉解表、清热解毒的功效。甲流患者表现为高热，微恶风寒，无汗，或有汗而汗出不畅，头痛，咽痛，咳嗽，口渴，舌尖偏红等症状时，可以选用银翘散。

麻杏石甘汤出自医圣张仲景的《伤寒论》，由麻黄、苦杏仁、石膏、甘草 4 味中药组成，具有辛凉解表、清肺平喘的功效。适用于发热持续，咳嗽喘急，鼻煽，口渴，有汗或无汗的甲流患者。临床上，银翘散和麻杏石甘汤常合方使

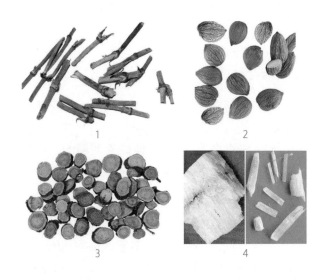

麻杏石甘汤组成药物图
1. 麻黄；2. 苦杏仁；
3. 甘草；4. 生石膏。

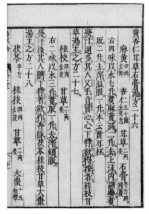
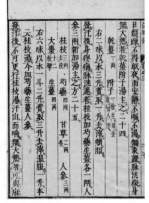

麻杏石甘汤条文

用。中国工程院王辰院士领衔开展的一项银翘散联合麻杏石甘汤治疗甲流的随机对照临床研究，共纳入 410 例甲流患者。研究发现，与单独应用奥司他韦相比，银翘散合麻杏石甘汤干预 5 天能显著缩短发热时间。在服用方法上，通常采用中药饮片水煎服，每日 1 剂，早晚各服 1 次。

参考文献

WANG C, CAO B, LIU Q Q, et al. Oseltamivir compared with the Chinese traditional therapy maxingshigan-yinqiaosan in the treatment of H1N1 influenza: a randomized trial[J]. Ann Intern Med, 2011,155(4):217-225.

第二节
心血管系统疾病

一、心血管系统疾病概述

心血管疾病是一类涉及心脏和血管的疾病，心血管疾病包括冠心病、高血压、心律失常、心力衰竭、心肌炎、心脏瓣膜病、心肌病等。心血管疾病的发生与多种危险因素密切相关，包括：高血压、吸烟、糖尿病、缺乏运动、肥胖、高脂血症等。心血管疾病已成为严重危害人民健康和生命的疾病，具有高死亡率、高致残率特征。

近 30 年来，西医学在心血管疾病的一级和二级预防上取得长足进步，包括针对冠心病的二级预防、介入治疗、冠状动脉旁路移植术治疗等，针对高血压的五大类降压药、新型降压药物研发以及经皮肾动脉交感神经消融术治疗，针对高脂血症的依折麦布、PCSK9 抑制剂等，针对心力衰竭的新型药物沙库巴曲缬沙坦钠片、左西孟旦等。然而，我国的心血管疾病（主要是冠心病、脑卒中等）死亡率、发病率、患病率均呈现上升趋势。目前，我国心血管疾病死亡率居于所有疾病死亡率之首，大约每 5 例死亡中就有 2 例死于心血管疾病。且在卫生经济学上，从 1980 年以来，我国心脑血管疾病患者出院人次数和医疗费用不断增加，2000 年以后增加迅速。心血管疾病已成为全球重大公共卫生问题。

然而，我们发现联合治疗带来的副作用以及不耐受问题，极大地限制了临床疗效。尤其是部分老年患者中存在阿司匹林抵抗，氯吡格雷抵抗，继发性硝酸甘油失效，利尿剂抵抗，他汀导致肝功能升高、肌痛，单硝酸异山梨酯导致的头痛，降压药导致的性功能下降等难题，严重地困扰了广大患者。同时，我们在临床上还发现，在部分人群中，运用中医药能够使得部分心血管疾病患者获益，不仅能改善临床症状，减少发作频次，减轻不良反应，甚至部分患者还可达到停减西药目标（医师指导下）。因此，在这里，我们将重点介绍冠心病、高血压、心律失常、心力衰竭、心肌炎、心肌病的中医药临床治疗思路与方法。

二、心血管系统疾病各论

1. 冠心病

冠心病是指由冠状动脉血管发生动脉粥样硬化进而导致血管腔狭窄或阻塞，引起心肌缺血、缺氧或坏死而导致的心脏病。世界卫生组织（WHO）将冠心病分为 5 大类：无症状心肌缺血、心绞痛、心肌梗死、缺血性心力衰竭（缺血性心脏病）和猝死。

在临床症状上，主要表现为体力活动、情绪激动后心前区疼痛加重，以绞痛、压榨痛、憋闷感为主。胸痛可向左肩、臂，甚至小指和无名指放射，也可放射到颈部、下颌、牙齿、腹部等，休息或含服硝酸甘油后缓解。然而，也有部分患者症状并不典型，仅表现为心前区不适、心悸或乏力，或以胃肠道症状为主，甚至部分糖尿病患者无任何不适症状。

在临床诊断上，需结合临床症状，辅助检查发现心肌缺血或冠脉阻塞证据，以及心肌损伤标志物。最常用的检查方法包括心电图、运动平板试验、核素心肌显像、冠状动脉造影等。

在西医学治疗上，包括戒烟限酒，低脂低盐饮食，适当体育锻炼，控制体重等生活习惯改变；抗血小板、抗凝、β受体阻滞剂、硝酸酯类、他汀类等药物治疗；介入治疗（血管内球囊扩张成形术和支架植入术）、外科冠状动脉旁路移植术等。

虽然西医学在诊断与治疗上取得了长足进步，然而仍然有部分患者胸痛、胸闷缓解不明显，且部分患者存在阿司匹林抵抗、不耐受硝酸酯类药物带来的头痛、不耐受他汀导致的肌肉疼痛等难题。部分患者会主动寻求中医药治疗，这在老年患者中尤其常见。

在中医学中，冠心病属于"胸痹心痛"范畴。在病因上，本病的发生多与寒邪内侵，饮食失调，情志失节，劳倦内伤，年迈体虚等因素有关。在病机上，存在虚与实这两种情况。虚证主要因心脉失养，不荣则痛，而实证则因瘀阻心脉，不通则痛。

在现代临床中，经典名方瓜蒌薤白半夏汤和中成药麝香保心丸运用尤其普遍。瓜蒌薤白半夏汤出自汉代医圣张仲景的《金匮要略》，由瓜蒌、薤白、姜半夏3味中药组成，具有通阳散结，祛痰宽胸功效。古人虽然不知道冠心病是什么原因导致的，但是在中医理论中，这就是因为痰浊邪气堵塞经络导致的胸阳痹阻不通。这种认识与西医学对冠心病的病理机制的认识有异曲同工之妙。而现代药理学研究也发现，本方具有保护心肌细胞、改善心功能、降脂、减轻动脉粥样硬化病变等作用。

中成药麝香保心丸是由复旦大学附属华山医院心内科戴瑞鸿教授，在宋代经典名方苏合香丸的基础上，运用现代药理学研究方法，对有效成分逐一进行筛选研发而成。该药具有芳香温通，益气强心功效，可用于气滞血瘀所致的冠心病。迄今为止，麝香保心丸已在临床运用近40年。特别是2021年发表在《中华医学杂志（英文版）》（*Chinese Medical Journal*）的 MUST 研究，备受关注，更是证实了麝香保心丸的临床价值。该研究由葛均波院士牵头，全国22个省、自治区和直辖市的97家三级医院参与，共纳入稳定型冠心病患者2673名，随访2年。研究表明，在阿司匹林和他汀类药物治疗基础上，与安慰剂组相比，加用麝香保心丸后，主要心血管不良事件（MACE）发生风险降低26.9%。此外，在持续用药18个月后，K-M曲线逐渐分离，且分离程度逐渐加大，显示出长期有效性和安全性。长期服用麝香保心丸，能够显著改善心绞痛稳定性和发作频率评分，这也表明麝香保心丸可有效缓解冠心病患者的临床症状，显著提升生活质量。本品味苦、辛凉，有麻舌感，为黑褐色有光泽的水丸，破碎后断面为棕黄色。服法为每次2丸，一日3次；或心绞痛症状发作时服用。

参考文献

GE J B, FAN W H, ZHOU J M, et al. Efficacy and safety of Shexiang Baoxin pill (MUSKARDIA) in patients with stable coronary artery disease: a multicenter, double-blind, placebo-controlled phase IV randomized clinical trial[J]. Chin Med J (Engl), 2020, 134(2): 185-192.

2. 高血压

高血压是指以体循环动脉血压增高为主要特征（收缩压≥140mmHg和舒张压≥90mmHg），可伴有心、脑、肾等重要靶器官的功能或器质性损害的一组临床综合征。高血压是临床最常见的慢性疾病，也是心脑血管病最重要的危险因素之一。随着年龄的增加，血压逐渐上升。我国现有高血压患者2.45亿人，高血压已成为我国重大公共卫生问题。

在临床症状上，高血压的症状因人而异，早期可无任何不适症状，很多年轻患者仅在体检时发现血压升高。临床常见症状包括头晕、头痛、项僵、疲劳、心悸、注意力不集中、记忆力减退、肢体麻木等。上述不适会在劳累、精神紧张、情绪波动后加重，在休息后症状减轻。

在临床诊断上，依据病史、体格检查和实验室检查结果即可确诊。本病分为原发性高血压与继发性高血压，两者之间需鉴别。继发性高血压病因包括肾实质性疾病、肾动脉狭窄、原发性醛固酮增多症、嗜铬细胞瘤等。

在临床治疗上，主要目标为血压达标，最终目的则是最大限度地减少心、脑血管疾病发生率和死亡率。治疗方式包括改善生活方式及药物治疗等。改善生活方式包括控制体重、低盐低脂饮食、补充钙和钾盐、运动、戒烟、限酒、减轻精神压力。常用的五大类降压药包括：利尿药、β受体阻滞剂、钙通道阻滞剂、血管紧张素转换酶抑制剂、血管紧张素Ⅱ受体阻滞剂。

虽然西医学在高血压的药物治疗上取得长足进步，然而，目前仍然存在"三高""三低""三不"现象，防治形势依然严峻。临床发现，部分患者虽然血压达标，但头晕头痛不适仍在。也有部分患者因长期服药、联合治疗等导致性功能下降、腰膝酸软、四肢无力、体力下降，严重降低了服药依从性。目前，中医药治疗高血压的整体调节优势已经受到国际权威杂志关注。

在中医学中，高血压属于"头痛""眩晕"范畴。在病因上，本病的发生多与情志失调、饮食不节、劳倦内伤、体虚久病等有关。在病机上，高血压与气血亏虚、肾精不足致脑髓空虚，清窍失养，或肝阳上亢、痰火上逆、瘀血阻窍而扰动清窍有关。

在现代临床中，经典名方天麻钩藤饮和中成药松龄血脉康胶囊运用尤其普遍。天麻钩藤饮出自近代医家胡光慈《中医内科杂病证治新义》，全方由天麻、钩藤、生决明、栀子、黄芩、川牛膝、桑寄生、杜仲、首乌藤、茯神、益母草组成。该方具有平肝息风、清热活血、滋补肝肾之效，主治肝阳偏亢，风阳上扰证。我们发现，本方可以广泛应用于高血压肝阳上亢证，针对病程较短或未服用降压药物干预的初发高血压、青年高血压患者效果更佳，同时也适用于3级高血压、高血压危象、高血压急症等急重症。2020年，上海瑞金医院王继光教授团队在 *Circulation* 杂志上发表了一项随机安慰剂对照临床试验，共纳入251名隐匿性高血压患者。隐匿性高血压是指诊室血压＜140/90 mmHg，但动态血压监测日间收缩压135～150mmHg或舒张压85～95 mmHg。研究显示，天麻钩藤颗粒组44.4%的患者日间血压降幅≥10/5 mmHg，中成药天麻钩藤颗粒对隐匿性高血压有效，而且治疗过程中未出现不良反应。

中成药松龄血脉康胶囊由鲜松叶与葛根以6∶1比例混合，再加辅料珍珠层粉制成，具有平肝潜阳，镇心安神功效。2022年，*Cardiovascular Quality and Outcomes* 杂志在线发表一项松龄血脉康胶囊治疗原发性高血压（1级）的随机、双盲、双模拟、多中心临床研究，共纳入628名1级高血压患者，并以1∶1的比例将患者随机分入松龄血脉康组和对照药物组，疗程8周。结果表明，在降低舒张压方面，松龄血脉康胶囊非劣于对照药物；在降低收缩压及改善24小时动态血压方面，两者效果相当；在降低血清总胆固醇和改善高血压症状（尤其是肝阳上亢相关症状）上，松龄血脉康胶囊显著优于对照药物。

另外，太极拳、八段锦、气功、瑜伽等运动，针刺疗法以及灸法、推拿、拔罐、浴足等其他疗法在高血压中运用极为广泛。大量国内外研究发现，太极拳不仅有助于降压，改善头痛头晕症状，还可调节血管内皮功能，降低炎症介质表达，改善动脉硬化，降低心率，降低心肌耗氧，改善心肌重构，改善糖脂代谢。中国健身气功协会建议在社区推广八段锦，改善高血压患者血压水平、临床症状及生活质量，对提高心脏病患者的活动耐量有益。研究发现，练习八段锦 3 个月至 1 年，收缩压可降低 13mmHg，舒张压可降低 6.13mmHg。

作为中医药疗法中应用最广泛的非药物疗法，针刺不仅可改善高血压患者临床症状，而且能平稳降压，减少并发症及靶器官损害。在辨证选穴方面，《高血压诊疗专家共识》指出常用降压穴位包括太冲、行间、涌泉、阳陵泉、三阴交、足三里、丰隆、太溪、曲池。石学敏院士也发现，针刺可有效控制血压，且起效迅速，降压持续性较好。

推拿可以疏通经络、调和气血，同样可以用于治疗高血压。有研究发现，在常规降压药基础上，推拿治疗 20 天至 4 个月，收缩压可以降低 6.92mmHg，舒张压可以降低 3.63mmHg，眩晕、头痛、腰膝酸软、五心烦热的临床症状得以明显改善。

浴足也是中医外治法之一，通过温水的热性物理刺激以行气活血、疏通经络，加快血液循环。国医大师邓铁涛教授喜欢用浴足的办法辅助治疗高血压，尤其针对肝火亢盛、阴虚阳亢证高血压患者，每日浴足 2 次，不仅可改善血压水平，还能改善头晕症状。应注意的是，在浴足过程中，要注意保暖，避风寒，同时有皮肤疾病、烧烫伤等患者不宜浴足。

参考文献

ZHANG D Y, CHENG Y B, GUO Q H, et al. Treatment of masked hypertension with a Chinese herbal formula[J]. Circulation, 2020, 142: 1821-1830.

LAI X, DONG Z, WU S, et al. Efficacy and safety of Chinese herbal medicine compared with losartan for mild essential hypertension: a randomized, multicenter, double-blind, noninferiority trial[J]. Circulation: Cardiovascular Quality and Outcomes, 2022, 15(3): e007923. doi: 10.1161/CIRCOUTCOMES. 121. 007923.

熊兴江，王阶. 论高血压病的中医认识及经典名方防治策略 [J]. 中医杂志，2011, 52(23): 1985-1989.

3. 心律失常

很多患者都可能有过心慌的感觉，在医学上这很有可能就是心律失常。心律失常是指心脏冲动的起源部位、心搏频率和节律以及冲动传导的任一异常而言。在病因上，可以由各种器质性心血管疾病、药物中毒、电解质和酸碱平衡失调等因素引起，也可出现在没有任何基础疾病的自主神经功能紊乱患者中。

按心律失常发作时心率的快慢，可以分为快速性和缓慢性心律失常两大类，前者见于期前收缩、心动过速、心房颤动（简称房颤）和心室颤动等；后者以窦性缓慢性心律失常和各种传导阻滞为常见。

在临床诊断上，主要依靠心电图，但也有相当一部分患者根据病史和体征就能作出初步诊断。可以详细追问患者发作的时候，心率快不快，节律乱不乱，是否有漏搏感等，发作时有没有低血压、昏厥、抽搐、心绞痛等，这些都有助于判断心律失常的性质。

在治疗上，有药物和非药物这两种类型。非药物疗法包括射频导管消融术治疗快速性心律失常、植入永久性心脏起搏器治疗缓慢性心律失常、埋藏式心脏复律除颤器治疗恶性室性心律失常等。但非药物疗法对技术设备要求高，且治疗费用相对昂贵。治疗心律失常的常用药物包括钠、钾、钙通道阻滞剂和 β 受体阻滞剂这几类，值得注意的是，这些药物往往疗效不佳，且"治"心律失常的药物很多具有"致"心律失常、心功能损害、诱发心力衰竭、甲状腺功能减退、肝功能损害等副作用，甚至增加死亡率，且对于缓慢性心律失常更是没有可以长期应用的西药。近年来，中医药治疗心律失常的临床价值逐渐受到患者认可。

在中医学中，心律失常属于"心悸"范畴。在病因上，本病的发生多与体虚久病禀赋不足，素体虚弱，或久病失养，劳欲过度，饮食劳倦，嗜食膏粱厚味，平素心虚胆怯，突遇惊恐或情怀不适，悲哀过极，感受外邪风寒湿邪气，药物中毒等有关。在病机上，心律失常与血阴阳亏虚，心失所养，或痰饮瘀血阻滞，心脉不畅有关。

在现代临床中，常用经典名方炙甘草汤、温胆汤和中成药参松养心胶囊。炙甘草汤出自汉代医著《伤寒论》，在古代这张处方又叫复脉汤，就是能让紊乱的脉律恢复正常的意思。在原文中，炙甘草汤用于治疗脉结代、心动悸，主要功效为益气滋阴，通阳复脉。目前临床上已经将该处方广泛用于室性期前收缩、房性期前收缩、房颤等一系列心律失常患者，同时伴有心律不齐、心悸、气短、舌红或舌光、色淡、少津。除此之外，我们发现，本方还能用于部分房颤患者的转窦且不发生血栓事件。

温胆汤出自宋代的《三因极一病证方论》，由半夏、竹茹、枳实、陈皮、甘草、茯苓组成，具有理气化痰，和胃利胆功效。现在临床上大多用来主治胆郁痰扰证，患者可能表现为胆怯易惊，容易心慌心悸，尤其是容易被外来的声音吓一跳，还会伴有心烦不眠，夜多异梦，噩梦纷纭，恶心头痛，眩晕，癫痫，苔白腻，脉弦滑等表现。心律失常患者，很多都会有上述的症状。中国中医科学院广安门医院院内制剂温胆宁心颗粒就是出自于温胆汤，临床运用非常广泛，深受患者欢迎。

参松养心胶囊是由中国工程院吴以岭院士基于中医"气-阴阳-五行"思想，提出由"调"致"平"的整合调律新策略研制而成。参松养心胶囊由人参、麦冬、山茱萸、丹参、酸枣仁、桑寄生、赤芍、土鳖虫、甘松、黄连、南五味子、龙骨等组成，具有益气养阴，活血通络，清心安神的功效，可用于治疗冠心病室性期前收缩，经中医辨证属于气阴两虚，心络瘀阻证。患者可以表现为心悸不安，气短乏力、动则加剧，胸部闷痛，失眠多梦，盗汗，神倦懒言。目前，参松养心胶囊已完成室性期前收缩、阵发性房颤、缓慢性心律失常、轻中度心功能不全伴室性期前收缩、窦性心动过缓伴室性期前收缩 5 种疾病的多中心随机双盲临床试验的循证研究。参松养心胶囊可以调节多离子和非离子通道，同时能调节自主神经，改善窦房结功能，促进心肌的电传导，改善心肌供血，抑制心室重构，保护心脏功能。该药的用法用量为口服，一次 2 ~ 4 粒，一日 3 次。

参考文献

熊兴江. 基于现代病理生理及 CCU 急危重症病例的炙甘草汤方证溯源及其复律、转窦、止血、升血小板、补虚临床运用 [J]. 中国中药杂志，2019，44（18）：3842-3860.

4. 心力衰竭

临床上见到很多冠心病、心脏瓣膜病患者，在某一次"感冒受凉"后出现喘憋加重，双下肢水肿，呼吸困难，去医院检查后确诊为"心力衰竭"。心力衰竭是指由于心脏的收缩功能或舒张功能发生障碍，不能将静脉回心血量充分排出心脏，导致静脉系统血液瘀积，动脉系统血液灌注不足，从而引起心脏循环障碍症候群。心力衰竭并不是一个独立的疾病，而是心脏疾病发展的终末阶段。大部分心力衰竭都是从左心衰竭开始，即表现为肺循环瘀血。本病发病率高，五年存活率与恶性肿瘤相似。

在病因上，几乎所有的心血管疾病最终都会导致心力衰竭的发生，包括冠状动脉硬化、高血压、心瓣膜疾病等。在心脏疾病基础上，心力衰竭的突然加重，大多存在诱发因素。常见诱因包括：呼吸道感染，风湿活动，快速性心律失常如房颤，阵发性心动过速，妊娠、分娩、输液过多过快、过多摄入钠盐等导致心脏负荷增加，洋地黄中毒，过度的体力活动和情绪激动。其他如肺栓塞、贫血、乳头肌功能不全等也会引起心力衰竭。一到秋冬季节，大量慢性心力衰竭的患者在受凉后就会喘憋加重，合并肺部感染，前来住院治疗。因此，如何控制好感染，注意保暖对于心力衰竭患者尤为关键。

在临床症状上，呼吸困难是左心衰最常见的临床症状，可表现为劳力性呼吸困难、端坐呼吸、阵发性夜间呼吸困难等。还可以见到运动耐力下降、乏力等。在右心衰时，患者还可以出现腹部或腿部水肿。大量患者是因为突然发现下肢水肿，或者体力下降前来就诊。

在临床诊断上，根据既往有冠心病、高血压等基础心血管疾病的病史，有休息或运动时出现呼吸困难、乏力、下肢水肿的临床症状，有心动过速、呼吸急促、肺部啰音、心脏杂音、超声心动图、NT-proBNP 水平升高等客观证据，就可以做出诊断。

在临床治疗上，目前已从利尿、强心、扩张血管等短期血流动力学/药理学治疗方案，转变为以神经内分泌抑制剂为主的长期、修复性策略。虽然西医学在治疗上取得长足进步，但仍然有部分患者心力衰竭反复发作，对利尿剂反应弱，甚至出现利尿剂抵抗，喘憋、水肿改善不理想。

在中医学中，心力衰竭属于"水肿""喘证"范畴。中医学认为，这种情况与肾阳虚衰，元气不足，心血痹阻，水饮内停，瘀血内阻有关，为本虚标实，虚实夹杂之证。如果不能得以救治，患者长期反复喘憋、水肿，容易导致喘脱重症。这种在本质上属于阳气大虚的疾病，已经属古代的"虚劳"病。值得注意的是，在西医学中，只有针对疾病的治疗理念与方法，而缺乏针对虚证的补虚概念。中医学的虚证与补虚是中医药针对部分西医学疾病诊疗方案的有效补充与完善。我们发现，顽固性心力衰竭、扩张型心肌病、缺血性心肌病、心脏瓣膜病等心血管疾病属于传统的"虚劳"范畴。在这种情况下，我们推荐运用膏方调理慢性心力衰竭。

膏方，又称膏滋、煎膏，是将中药饮片经过反复煎煮，去渣取汁，经过蒸发、浓缩，添加辅料，收膏等过程而制成的半流体状剂型。膏方多为"虚证""虚劳"而设，现今临床多将膏方用于"治未病"，滋补调养，养生寿老，防衰延年，以及预防和治疗慢性疾病。在治疗重症心力衰竭、扩张型心肌病、缺血性心肌病、心脏瓣膜病等方面，长期服食补益膏方，不仅能够有效减轻症状，提高生活质量，还能改善心脏结构与功能，减少利尿剂用量，减少住院次数，达到二级预防目的。在膏方里面，我们经常用党参、白术、黄芪等健脾益气中药，能够较好改善心力衰竭患者出现的乏力、喘憋等症状。我们曾经治疗过一例心脏瓣膜病，三尖瓣下移畸形（Ebstein 畸形），慢性心力衰竭，心功能Ⅳ级（NYHA 分级）患者，NT-proBNP 为 12539pg/ml，心力衰竭频繁发作，一年住院 6 次，反复发作，反复住院，治之以温阳益气膏方，随访 2 年未再住院。

中药治疗心力衰竭的经验值得关注。

参考文献

熊兴江，尤虎，苏克雷. 中药补益膏方对重症心衰"虚劳"的二级预防 [J]. 中国中药杂志，2019，44（18）：3903-3907.

5. 病毒性心肌炎

在门诊经常会遇到一些小朋友，误以为得了感冒，一直到出现严重的胸闷、心慌等不适才会来医院就诊，在做心电图和抽血查心肌酶时，发现结果异常，直至最终被确诊为"病毒性心肌炎"。

病毒性心肌炎是病毒感染引起的心肌局限性或弥漫性的急性或慢性炎症病变，属于感染性心肌疾病。在病毒流行感染期，约有 5% 患者会出现心肌炎，也可散在发病。其中，柯萨奇病毒 B 组病毒是最主要的病毒。

在临床表现上，病毒性心肌炎的严重程度取决于心肌病变的部位和广泛程度。轻者可不表现为任何不适，严重的可出现心力衰竭、心源性休克和猝死。在本病发病前 1~3 周，通常会有上呼吸道或肠道感染的病史，部分患者会出现发热、浑身酸痛、咽痛、倦怠乏力、恶心呕吐、腹泻等症状，继而出现胸闷、胸痛、心前区隐痛、心慌、头晕、呼吸困难、下肢水肿，甚至发生阿–斯综合征；极少数患者会表现为心力衰竭或心源性休克。

在临床诊断上，结合前驱感染病史，临床表现，心电图以及心肌损伤标志物就可以考虑该疾病诊断。但是本病确诊有赖于心内膜心肌活检。

虽然能够明确诊断该病，但当前尚缺乏特异性治疗手段，仅以营养心肌、对症治疗等为主。部分患者会在急性期主动寻求中医药治疗，以加快康复。门诊也有不少因心肌炎后胸闷、心慌而来就诊的，服用中药有助于缓解胸闷、心慌的临床不适症状。

在中医学中，病毒性心肌炎属于"心悸""胸痹""温病"等范畴，多与外感温热邪毒，由表入里，损伤心脏有关。外感温热邪气，很容易出现耗气伤阴。因此，临床所见，心之气阴两伤为病毒性心肌炎的发病之本。

经典名方炙甘草汤与生脉散均为临床常用的治疗病毒性心肌炎的代表性方剂。炙甘草汤出自于《伤寒论》，原文主治"脉结代，心动悸"。这提示，在古代这就是用于治疗脉律不齐，心慌心悸，倦怠乏力，舌光红，少苔，或无苔，或舌质干而瘦小的处方。而病毒性心肌炎患者，很容易合并出现上述证候。因为这张处方对于改善心慌心悸有显著功效，常被认为是病毒性心肌炎的专病专方。岳美中先生也喜欢用这张方子治疗病毒性心肌炎。

生脉散也是中医学的经典名方，由人参、麦冬、五味子组成，属于补益剂，具有益气生津，敛阴止汗功效。生脉散可以主治气阴两伤证，患者表现为汗多神疲，体倦乏力，气短懒言，咽干口渴，舌干红少苔，脉虚数就可以用这张处方。部分病毒性心肌炎患者在急性期或恢复期会表现为走路乏力，这就属于生脉散的典型适应证。中成药生脉饮口服液就出自于生脉散这张处方。

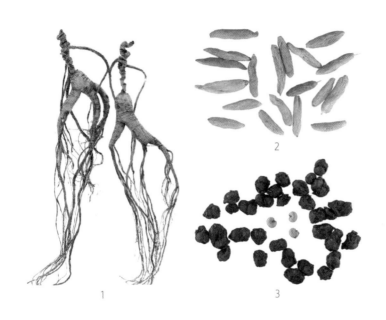

生脉散组成药物图
1. 人参；2. 麦冬；3. 五味子。

在预后方面，大多数患者经治疗后都能痊愈，仅有极少数患者在急性期出现严重心律失常、急性心力衰竭和心源性休克死亡。如果不注意休息，甚至耽误治疗，部分患者会发展成为扩张型心肌病。在临床上，我们见过反复咽痛，误认为感冒，直至胸闷心慌，喘憋不能平卧后方来就诊，确诊为扩张型心肌病的年轻患者，殊为可惜。

6. 心肌病

心肌病是由不同病因引起的心脏机械和电活动的异常，表现为心室的肥厚或扩张。严重的心肌病能导致死亡或心力衰竭。心肌病通常分为原发性心肌病和继发性心肌病，其中原发性心肌病包括扩张型心肌病、肥厚型心肌病、限制型心肌病、致心律失常性右室心肌病和未定型心肌病。继发性心肌病指心肌病是全身性疾病的一部分。

在病因上，心肌病的发生与很多因素密切相关。原发性心肌病的发病原因不明，继发性心肌病主要与感染、代谢疾病、内分泌疾病、缺血、过敏等因素有关。

在临床症状上，各种心肌病症状表现有差异。扩张型心肌病多缓慢起病，有时可达10年以上，在中年人中常见。临床常以气短和水肿为主要症状。最初可在劳累后出现乏力气短，以后可在轻度活动时出现气短。肥厚型心肌病可以没有任何不适，也可以表现为心悸、劳力性呼吸困难、心前区闷痛、易疲劳、晕厥甚至猝死。

在临床诊断上，结合病史、查体、心电图、X线、超声心动图、冠状动脉造影、放射性核素心室造影等可得出诊断。

在临床治疗上，主要包括针对病因治疗和对症治疗。值得注意的是，心肌病一旦形成，则会出现心脏收缩或舒张功能的改变，大多难以逆转。尤其是在射血分数低于30%时，虽然部分患者可能胸闷憋气临床症状不明显，但存在较高的潜在猝死风险。心肌病患者大都会积极寻求中医药治疗，以改善症状，改善生活质量，减少死亡率。

中医学认为，心肌病属于"水肿""喘证""胸痹"等范畴。在病因上，素体心气不足，或心肾阳虚为内因；而外邪侵袭、过度劳累，久病失调等则为外因。一般而言，本病为本虚标实。

在临床中，经典名方真武汤使用频率极高。真武汤出自汉代《伤寒论》，由茯苓、芍药、生姜、附子、白术组成，具有温阳利水功效。真武汤主治阳虚水泛证。心肌病患者出现的喘憋不能平卧，双下肢水肿，心慌心悸，头晕目眩，站立不稳，小便不利，小便量少，舌质淡胖，边有齿痕，舌苔白滑，脉沉细等，都属于真武汤的主治范畴。我们发现，部分患者在长期服用真武汤后，射血分数能够得以提升。曾经治疗过一例扩张性心肌病患者，射血分数为21%，行冠状动脉造影排除冠心病，住院期间患者被告知可以考虑心脏再同步化治疗，但家属因为费用极高而拒绝。患者经真武汤治疗2年后，射血分数提升至48%，心功能得到改善，且避免了心脏再同步化治疗的沉重经济负担。

参考文献

熊兴江. 《伤寒论》与急危重症——基于CCU重症病例及中西医结合诠释经典条文内涵、经方剂量与六经实质 [J]. 中国中药杂志, 2018, 43（12）: 2413-2430.

第三节
消化系统疾病

一、消化系统疾病概述

老百姓常说"能吃是福"，但只是"能吃"还不够，吃进去的食物还得能被顺利地消化、吸收，最后还要能把垃圾废物通过粪便排出去，才算是圆满。所有这一切，都取决于我们消化系统的功能是否正常，一旦这条"生产线"的任何一环出现故障，就患上了所谓的消化系统疾病。

在西医学中，消化系统疾病是一组系统疾病的统称，常见的有胃炎、消化性溃疡、胃癌、胃食管反流病、食管癌、溃疡性结肠炎等。临床表现除恶心、呕吐、反酸、腹痛、腹泻、便血等消化系统本身症状外，也常伴有其他系统或全身性症状。在临床诊断上，除主诉外，还需要结合实验室检查、内镜检查，腹部 B 超、腹平片、腹盆部 CT 或 MR 等影像学检查，以及病理活检结果，方能确诊。

在临床治疗上，常用治疗手段包括药物治疗、内镜治疗、手术治疗、放化疗和免疫靶向治疗等。然而，临床发现，仍有部分患者症状改善不理想，依然存在厌食、恶心、纳差、腹泻等明显不适，进而寻求中医药治疗。中医学在改善消化系统疾病相关症状，调理体质，提高生活质量等方面具有显著优势。

根据症状，消化系统疾病属于"胃痛""腹痛""噎膈""泄泻""便秘"等范畴，其病位在脾、胃、肠。本节将重点讨论中医药在功能性消化不良、胃食管反流病、胃炎、便秘、溃疡性结肠炎、慢性腹泻方面的认识与治疗。

二、消化系统疾病各论

1. 功能性消化不良

功能性消化不良是临床上最常见的一种功能性胃肠病，是由胃和十二指肠功能紊乱所致。患者常表现为"吃一点儿就饱了""正常食量，但是饭后饱胀难受"、恶心、食欲下降、打嗝、中上腹部"火辣辣地疼"……但是去医院检查，却没有发现器质性病变。

在临床诊断上，首先要确定患者近期没有消瘦、贫血、呕血、黑便、腹部肿块、黄疸等提示器质性病变的症状和体征，排除消化道器质性疾病，再结合具体消化不良症状、血液生化、胃肠镜等检查结果，最终明确诊断。

在临床治疗上，以对症药物治疗和生活、饮食习惯调整为主。然而，仍有部分患者在服药及改变生活习惯后，症状仍反复发作，并由此而产生失眠、焦虑、抑郁等问题。

中医药在治疗功能性消化不良方面有着一定的临床优势。在中医学中，功能性消化不良属于"胃痛""痞满""呃逆"等范畴。在病因上，多由感受外邪、饮食不当、情志不遂诱发；在病机上，多与脾胃纳运失司、升降失调有关。

在临床治疗上，常用四磨汤口服液及针刺疗法。四磨汤出自宋代严用和的《济生方》，由天台乌药、沉香、人参、槟榔 4 味中药组成，具有顺气降逆，消积止痛功效。该方可以治疗食积气滞所导致的腹部胀满、疼痛、大便不畅等症状，还可治疗成年人的术后腹胀。功能性消化不良患者症见厌食、纳差、脘腹胀满、腹痛、便秘，可以服用本方。现在已将本方研制而成四磨汤口服液，用法用量为每次口服 20ml，每日 3 次，疗程一周。一项纳入了 27 项临床研究、共 2713 例消化不良患者的系统评价研究显示，四磨汤口服液不仅能缩短胃排空的时间，提高胃排空率，还能降低功能性消化不良的复发率。

除上述药物疗法外，针刺疗法也常用于缓解功能性消化不良症状。临床常用穴位包括上脘、中脘、下脘、内关、膻中、天枢、足三里、梁丘等，并在此基础上进行中医辨证选穴。一项纳入了 278 名功能性消化不良患者的随机对照临床研究显示，与假针灸组相比，每周 3 次，持续 4 周的针刺治疗能有效缓解饭后饱胀感、早饱、上腹胀三大主要症状，治疗结束后随访 12 周未见反复。

参考文献

HU Y, BAI Y, HUA Z, et al. Effect of Chinese patent medicine Si-Mo-Tang oral liquid for functional dyspepsia: a systematic review and meta-analysis of randomized controlled trials[J]. PLoS One, 2017, 12(2): e0171878.

YANG J W, WANG L Q, ZOU X, et al. Effect of acupuncture for postprandial distress syndrome: a randomized clinical trial[J]. Ann Intern Med, 2020, 172(12): 777-785.

2. 胃食管反流病

我们身边时常出现这样一些人，每次吃完饭后，别人都舒服地坐着、躺着，他们却坐立难安，反复抱怨说"胃里面火辣辣地疼""烧心""不敢打嗝，一打嗝就反酸水""酸水烧得嗓子难受、想咳嗽"……如果身边的亲朋好友出现上述不适症状，一定要警惕一种病——胃食管反流病。

胃食管反流病是一种由胃、十二指肠内容物反流入食管引起不适症状或并发症的疾病。正常情况下，胃十二指肠内容物是不会反流到食管里的。如果长期吸烟、饮酒，进食过饱，嗜食高糖、高脂肪、辛辣刺激性食物，或者长期服用某些刺激性药物，导致食管一过性松弛延长、食管蠕动异常、食管黏膜防御屏障破坏，胃十二指肠内容物就会"逆流而上"到食管。因为反流物中含有胃酸、胃蛋白酶之类的强酸性成分，故而会引起食管黏膜不同程度的损伤，甚至发生黏膜糜烂、溃疡。

在临床症状上，反流和烧心最为常见，也最典型。通常出现在餐后1小时左右，仰卧、弯腰、夜间睡眠时可加重。一些患者还会出现反酸、胸痛。还有部分患者还表现为咽部异物感、堵塞感，刺激性干咳或哮喘，甚至以此为首发症状就诊，呼吸科专科检查未见异常，最终确诊为胃食管反流病。

在临床诊断上，可予质子泵抑制剂（如奥美拉唑）试验性治疗，症状明显缓解的，可以初步诊断为本病。当然，还需结合胃镜、食管造影、24小时食管pH监测结果，并排除消化系统其他疾病和引起相关症状的其他系统疾病，方能确诊。

在临床治疗上，包括调整生活方式，药物治疗（抑酸药、促胃肠动力药、抗酸药），手术治疗等。然而，部分患者虽然长期口服西药治疗，但反酸、烧心症状持续存在，进而求助于中医药治疗。中医药在缓解胃食管反流病相关症状，减少复发频次，改善生活质量等方面，具有一定临床优势。

在中医学中，本病属于"吐酸"范畴。在病因上，多与饮食失节、起居不慎有关。在病机上，与肝气犯胃、胃失和降有关。

在临床治疗中，临床常用小柴胡汤和吴茱萸汤等经典名方。小柴胡汤出自医圣张仲景的《伤寒论》，由柴胡、黄芩、半夏、生姜、人参、大枣、甘草7味中药组成，具有和解少阳之功效。胃食管反流伴见口干口苦、胸骨后烧灼感、咽部不适、慢性咳嗽，或伴有食欲不振、心烦、恶心等，可选用小柴胡汤。根据 *World Journal of Gastroenterololy* 发表的一项临床研究显示，小柴胡汤不但能提高轻中度胃食管反流病患者食管下括约肌收缩力、减少无效吞咽，还能显著降低3个月内的复发率，其作用类似于质子泵抑制剂。

吴茱萸汤同样也是出自医圣张仲景的《伤寒论》，由吴茱萸、生姜、人参、大枣4味中药组成，具有温中补虚，降逆止呕功效。该方适用于食后恶心欲呕，或干呕，或呕吐酸水，或吐清冷稀水，伴有胸闷、胃部不适、头顶痛、怕冷、四肢凉、腹泻、烦躁等症状患者。一项纳入 90 例胃食管反流病患者的随机对照临床试验显示，与单用奥美拉唑相比，加用吴茱萸汤不仅能改善反流和烧心症状，且作用维持时间更长。

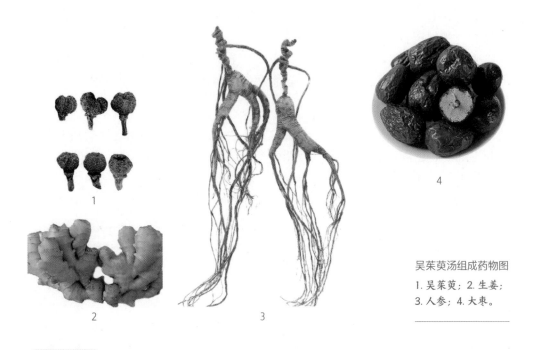

吴茱萸汤组成药物图
1. 吴茱萸；2. 生姜；
3. 人参；4. 大枣。

参考文献

XU L Y, YU B Y, CEN L S. New treatment for gastroesophageal reflux disease: Traditional Chinese medicine Xiaochaihu decoction[J]. World J Gastroenterol, 2022, 28(11): 1184-1186.

SHIH Y S, TSAI C H, LI T C, et al. Effect of wu zhu yu tang on gastroesophageal reflux disease: randomized, double-blind, placebo-controlled trial[J]. Phytomedicine, 2019, 56: 118-125.

3. 慢性胃炎

慢性胃炎是指由多种病因引起的慢性胃黏膜炎症病变。最常见的病因是幽门螺杆菌感染。此外，某些药物、酒精、自身免疫、年龄增长等也能诱发。大多数成年人的胃黏膜都会有轻微的浅表性炎症，但大多没有明显的不适。

在临床症状上，慢性胃炎常表现为中上腹不适、饱胀感、隐痛、钝痛、烧灼感、食欲不振、恶心、泛酸、嗳气等消化不良症状，但是缺乏特异性。病情严重的可见全身虚弱无力、厌食、贫血、体重下降、呕血、黑便等，甚至进展为胃癌。

在临床诊断上，胃镜和组织学检查是诊断的关键，仅凭临床表现并不能做出特异性诊断。

在临床治疗上，以药物干预为主。对于幽门螺杆菌阳性患者，常规采用"四联疗法"。此外，还包括对症治疗、生活和饮食习惯纠正等。多数患者经过上述干预措施后，症状可明显缓解。但仍有部分患者出现抗生素不耐受、停药后幽门螺杆菌再次阳性，以及在治疗过程中症状缓解不理想等难题，转而寻求中医的帮助。中医药在改善慢性胃炎的临床症状上具有一定疗效。

在中医学中，慢性胃炎属于"胃痛""痞满""呕吐"范畴。在病因上，与感受外邪、饮食失当、情志不节等有关。在病机上，多与脾胃功能失调，升降失司，胃气壅塞或胃气上逆有关。

在临床治疗上，常用小柴胡汤和黄连素片。小柴胡汤出自医圣张仲景的《伤寒论》，由柴胡、黄芩、半夏、生姜、人参、大枣、甘草7味中药组成，具有和解少阳之功效。本方适用于慢性胃炎患者，症见食欲不振、恶心、嗳气、中上腹饱胀感，或伴有口干、口苦、心烦等。实验研究证实，小柴胡汤不仅能有效抑制幽门螺杆菌，对于酒精引起的胃损伤，还显示出预防和胃保护作用。

黄连素片是最为大家熟知的治疗腹泻的药物之一，以其价格便宜、方便服用和携带而受到大众的青睐。黄连素，又称小檗碱，是从中药黄连中分离的一种季铵生物碱，是黄连的主要抗菌成分。除了治疗腹泻，黄连素片也常用于治疗慢性胃炎。黄连素片适用于症见中上腹部胀痛、呕吐，或伴有腹泻、口渴、目赤、牙痛、心烦、失眠的慢性胃炎患者。服用方法为成人每次1~3片，每日3次。临床研究证实，黄连素能有效治疗幽门螺杆菌引起的慢性萎缩性胃炎。

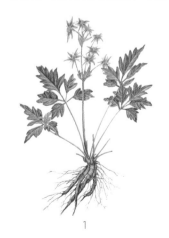

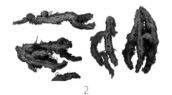

黄连植株及饮片图
1.原植物；2.黄连饮片。

1   2

参考文献

CHEN X, HU L J, WU H H, et al. Anti-*Helicobacter pylori* and anti-inflammatory effects and constituent analysis of modified Xiaochaihutang for the treatment of chronic gastritis and gastric ulcer[J]. Evid Based Complement Alternat Med, 2018, 2018: e6810369.

YANG T, WANG R L, LIU H H, et al. Berberine regulates macrophage polarization through IL-4-STAT6 signaling pathway in *Helicobacter pylori*-induced chronic atrophic gastritis[J]. Life Sci, 2021, 266: e118903.

4. 便秘

随着社会的发展，身边越来越多的人为便秘而苦恼。所谓的便秘，是指排便次数减少（每周排便少于3次）、粪便干硬和排便困难（排便费力、排出困难、排便不尽感、排便费时、需要手法辅助排便）。当便秘持续时间大于12周时，则称为慢性便秘。便秘不单单只是排便问题，长期反复的便秘还会使患者产生焦虑、烦躁、失眠等问题，严重影响生活质量和工作效率。

在病因上，其最常见的诱因包括不良的生活习惯和社会心理因素。前者包括进食过少，食物偏于精细化、高热量，蔬果摄入不足，久坐不动，不良的排便习惯等。社会心理因素主要是指人际关系、工作压力、突发事件等导致的自主神经功能紊乱、肠蠕动失调，或排便规律被打破。此外，某些疾病（如脑梗死、抑郁症、糖尿病、甲状腺功能减退）的并发症、某些药物的不良反应，以及手术，都有可能引发便秘。

在临床症状上，除了前面提到的一系列表现外，还常见下腹胀痛、食欲不振、疲乏无力、头晕、烦躁、失眠等，部分患者可因用力排便而导致肛门疼痛、肛裂、痔疮和肛门炎症。患者可以在左下腹部自行触及条索状物，即长时间贮留的粪便。

在临床诊断上，除了病史、临床症状、生活方式等，还需要结合腹部平片、胃肠镜、结肠传输试验等检查手段，方能明确便秘的病因和最终诊断。若相关辅助检查未提示有器质性病变，则诊断为功能性便秘。对于伴有便血、便潜血阳性、发热、贫血、呕吐、消瘦等症状的患者，应充分检查。

在临床治疗上，除了引导患者养成良好的生活和排便习惯外，药物治疗是常用手段，包括泻药、促胃肠动力药和调节肠道菌群的药物。我们发现，有部分患者在用药初期效果明显，但随着时间的推移，效果逐渐变差，甚至无效，出现继发性便秘，或服药时排便正常，一旦停药则便秘复发，均给患者带来极大的痛苦和心理负担，部分患者则会求助于中医药治疗。

在中医学中，"便秘"疾病和西医学所指的便秘在症状上符合。在病因上，多与感受外邪、饮食不节、情志不遂、病后体虚有关。在病机上，多属于邪滞大肠，腑气闭塞不通或肠失温润，推动无力，导致大肠传导功能失常。

在临床治疗上，常用经典名方麻子仁丸和针刺疗法。麻子仁丸出自医圣张仲景的《伤寒论》，由厚朴、枳实、火麻仁、白芍、大黄、杏仁、白蜜7味中药组成。麻子仁丸具有润肠泄热，行气通便之功效。该药能够治疗胃肠燥热型便秘，症见大便干结，腹胀腹痛，口干口臭，小便黄少灼热，或伴有面红身热，心烦不安，舌红苔黄。临床研究证实，麻子仁丸能够有效缓解功能性便秘，其作用机制与下调油酰胺水平，从而促进肠道蠕动有关。

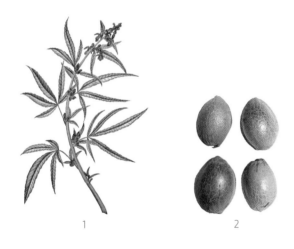

火麻仁原植物及饮片图
1.原植物; 2.火麻仁饮片。

临床上除了服药，针刺在治疗便秘方面具有不可忽视的疗效。我院针灸科刘志顺主任领衔开展的一项针对功能性便秘患者的临床研究显示，与假针刺组相比，在双侧天枢、腹结和上巨虚穴进行电针治疗，每次30分钟，疗程8周，治疗期间患者便秘症状明显缓解，自主排便次数增加，生活质量提高，且后续的随访中未见反复。其作用机制可能与副交感神经激活、结肠蠕动增强有关。上述研究发表于国际权威医学杂志 *Annals of Internal Medicine*，受到国际医学界关注。

参考文献

HUANG T, ZHAO L, LIN C Y, et al. Chinese herbal medicine (MaZiRenWan) improves bowel movement in functional constipation through down-regulating oleamide[J]. Front Pharmacol, 2020, 10: 1570.

LIU Z S, YAN S Y, WU J N, et al. Acupuncture for chronic severe functional constipation: a randomized trial[J]. Ann Intern Med, 2016,165 (11): 761-769.

5. 溃疡性结肠炎

溃疡性结肠炎是一种慢性非特异性肠道炎症性疾病，其病因尚未阐明，目前认为本病与环境因素、遗传因素、肠道微生态改变导致的肠道免疫失衡、肠黏膜屏障破坏以及肠黏膜持续炎症损伤有关。

在病变部位上，本病多从直肠开始，逆行向上累及结肠甚至末段回肠。病变呈连续性弥漫性分布，主要损害大肠黏膜层和黏膜下层，重症患者会累及肠壁全层，并发肠穿孔、中毒性巨结肠、腹腔脓肿等。

在临床表现上，本病的典型症状包括反复发作的腹泻、黏液脓血便和腹痛，一般呈发作期与缓解期交替。部分患者可伴有里急后重、腹胀、食欲减退、恶心呕吐、发热，以及消瘦、贫血等营养不良症状。也可见外周关节炎、口腔复发性溃疡、结节性红斑等肠外表现。

在临床诊断上，结肠镜是本病诊断和鉴别诊断的关键。必要时可取黏膜进行活检。若伴有发热、黏液脓血便严重，还需进行血常规、血沉、粪便病原学检查以进一步明确病情分期和判断是否合并感染。

在临床治疗上，以抗炎、免疫抑制和对症治疗为主，急重症患者必要时可进行手术治疗。一般轻症患者预后较好，但是对于老年患者以及发作频繁的患者，常见激素无效、激素依赖、胃肠道并发症、骨髓抑制等，导致病情反复发作。中医药治疗溃疡性结肠炎在改善临床症状、减少发作频次等方面具有一定优势。

在中医学中，溃疡性结肠炎属于"痢疾"范畴。在病因上，与外感时邪疫毒、饮食不洁有关。在病机上，多为邪蕴肠腑，气血凝滞，大肠脂膜血络受损，传导失司。

在临床治疗上，常用经典名方芍药汤和中成药黄连素片。芍药汤出自《素问病机气宜保命集》，由芍药、槟榔、大黄、黄芩、黄连、当归、肉桂、甘草、木香 9 味中药组成，具有清脏腑热，清热燥湿，调气和血之功效。主治湿热痢疾。适用于溃疡性结肠炎，症见腹痛，黏液脓血便、赤白相兼，伴有里急后重，肛门灼热，小便黄少、有灼热感，舌苔黄腻等。实验研究证实，芍药汤对溃疡性结肠炎具有保护作用，能够维护肠黏膜屏障的完整性，其作用机制可能与抑制 MKP1/NF-κB/NLRP3 通路有关。

黄连素片是广为人知的治疗腹泻的中成药。黄连素，又称小檗碱，是黄连的主要抗菌成分。黄连素适用于症见腹泻反复发作，大便味臭、可伴有黏液脓血，腹痛，里急后重，肛门灼热，口干口苦，心烦失眠，或伴有中上腹部不适，呕吐，反酸，嗳气的溃疡性结肠炎患者。黄连素的服用方法为成人每次 1~3 片，每日 3 次。实验研究证实，黄连素能激活 IL-25-ILC2-IL-13 免疫通路，促进肠干细胞分化，进而修复溃疡性结肠炎的肠黏膜屏障损害。

参考文献

WEI Y Y, FAN Y M, GA Y, et al. Shaoyao decoction attenuates DSS-induced ulcerative colitis, macrophage and NLRP3 inflammasome activation through the MKP1/NF-κB pathway[J]. Phytomedicine, 2021, 92: e153743.

XIONG X, CHENG Z, WU F, et al. Berberine in the treatment of ulcerative colitis: a possible pathway through Tuft cells[J]. Biomed Pharmacother, 2021, 134: e111129.

6. 慢性腹泻

慢性腹泻，是指排便次数增多（＞3 次 / 天），或大便量增加（＞200g/ 天），或大便稀薄（含水量＞85%），病程超过 4 周或长期反复发作。老百姓经常会说自己"动不动就闹肚子""我有老肠炎"……其实，慢性腹泻并不都是"肠炎"，从病因上讲，胃肠道、肝胆、胰腺以及其他诸多疾病都能导致慢性腹泻，这就是为什么有些患者按肠炎治疗多年，仍未见好转。

在发病机制与临床症状上，慢性腹泻可分为如下四种：渗透性腹泻、分泌性腹泻、渗出性腹泻和动力异常性腹泻。渗透性腹泻由进食不易消化的食物、食物不耐受或服用某些药物等，导致体液水分大量进入肠腔所致，一般禁食后腹泻减轻或停止。分泌性腹泻由肠黏膜分泌功能增强、吸收减弱，肠腔内水和电解质的净分泌量增加所致，特点为大便量多呈水样，无脓血，禁食不能缓解。渗出性腹泻，又称炎症性腹泻，由感染（细菌、病毒、寄生虫等）或非感染（自身免疫性疾病、肿瘤等）因素引起的肠黏膜炎症、坏死、渗出所致，其特点是粪便中含有渗出液或血液成分，甚至可见肉眼脓血。动力异常性腹泻由肠道蠕动过快，水和电解质吸收不足所致，其特征包括便急、不成形、伴有腹痛及肠鸣，常见的诱因包括受凉、糖尿病并发症、胃肠动力药，以及甲状腺功能亢进等代谢性疾病等。

在临床诊断上，最重要的是明确慢性腹泻的病因。需要结合病史，临床表现，以及腹部 B 超、胃肠镜、大便常规＋隐血、血液生化、肿瘤标志物等检查结果，方能明确病因、病变部位和最终诊断。

在临床治疗上，主要依靠药物疗法，包括对因治疗和对症治疗。常用药物有抗生素、益生菌、止泻药、抑制肠蠕动药等。然而，部分患者仍然存在症状缓解不明显，转而寻求中医药治疗。中医药在改善慢性腹泻症状，提高生活质量等方面具有一定疗效。

在中医学中，慢性腹泻属于"泄泻"范畴。在病因上，多与感受外邪、饮食不节、情志内伤、劳倦体虚有关。在病机上，多为脾虚湿盛、脾胃运化失职。

在临床治疗上，常用经典名方参苓白术散和附子理中丸。参苓白术散出自宋代《太平惠民和剂局方》，由白扁豆、白术、茯苓、甘草、桔梗、莲子、人参、砂仁、山药、薏苡仁 10 味中药组成，具有补脾胃，益肺气之功效。适用于慢性腹泻，症见腹泻反复发作，粪质稀薄，伴有腹胀，肠鸣音活跃，食欲不振，气短，咳嗽，胸闷，肢体乏力，形体消瘦者。本方已制成中成药制剂参苓白术颗粒，一般每次 1 袋（3g），一天 3 次。实验研究表明，参苓白术散能够缓解乳糖诱导的腹泻，其机制可能与调节肠道吸收功能和肠黏膜超微结构有关。

附子理中丸也出自宋代《太平惠民和剂局方》，由附子、人参、干姜、甘草、白术 5 味中药组成，具有温中健脾之功效。主治脾胃虚寒证。适用于症见腹泻反复发作，粪质稀薄，没有臭味或略有腥臭味，不伴有里急后重、肛门灼热，腹部冷痛，

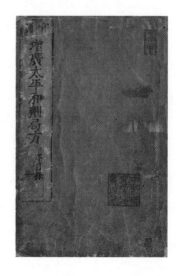

《增广太平惠民和剂局方》

中国中医科学院馆藏

腹胀，肠鸣音亢进，饮食不佳、喜热食，手脚冰凉，或伴有呕吐，嗳气，反酸等慢性腹泻患者。常规服法为一次1丸，一日2~3次。实验研究表明，附子理中丸治疗腹泻的机制可能与调节肠道菌群的多样性和群落结构，调节炎症和免疫系统有关。

参考文献

JI H J, KANG N, CHEN T, et al. Shen-ling-bai-zhu-san, a spleen-tonifying Chinese herbal formula, alleviates lactose-induced chronic diarrhea in rats[J]. J Ethnopharmacol, 2019, 231: 355-362.

ZHEN Z, XIA L, YOU H, et al. An integrated gut microbiota and network pharmacology study on Fuzi-Lizhong Pill for treating diarrhea-predominant irritable bowel syndrome[J]. Front Pharmacol, 2021, 12: e746923.

第四节
泌尿系统疾病

一、泌尿系统疾病概述

有的人早上起床时突然发现双眼睑肿得发亮了，如果有一点健康常识，可能就会想到查查尿常规，排查自己是不是得了肾病。我们曾经见过一位很干练的研究生，突然出现颜面部水肿，后来经诊断，明确为急性肾小球肾炎。

泌尿系统主要由肾脏、输尿管、膀胱、尿道及相关血管、神经组成。临床常见的泌尿系统疾病，包括肾小球肾炎、IgA 肾病、慢性肾衰竭、尿路感染、尿失禁等疾病。其临床表现多样，肾脏疾病可表现为血尿、蛋白尿、水肿、高血压、肾功能损害等，尿路感染可表现为尿频、尿急、尿痛、发热、腰痛及尿液性状异常改变等。

在治疗上，常用药物包括抗生素、利尿剂、激素、细胞毒类药物等。然而，泌尿系统疾病大多病情复杂，缠绵难愈，临床效果不尽如人意。患者不仅常常在面对如慢性肾衰竭这样的重大疾病时感到焦虑，如果在体检时发现了尿蛋白、尿潜血、轻度肌酐升高等，患者也会惴惴不安而四处求医问药，很多患者还会选择中医药治疗。

泌尿系统疾病属于中医"肾系"病证，归属于"水肿""淋证""尿浊""关格"等范畴。中医认为此类疾病病位在肾与膀胱，病因病机多与脾肾亏虚、气化失司，或湿热蕴结、水液运化失常等密切相关。在中医治疗上，常以补脾益肾或清热利湿为主要治疗原则，同时根据具体情况辨证论治。在各论中，我们将围绕急性肾小球肾炎、IgA 肾病、慢性肾衰竭、尿路感染、尿失禁，介绍中医药治疗特色与优势。

二、泌尿系统疾病各论

1. 急性肾小球肾炎

在临床上，我们经常见到一些患者，在患扁桃体炎、猩红热或脓疱疮后，突然出现颜面部或下肢水肿，并可能伴有蛋白尿、肉眼血尿及高血压等表现。这可能是感染后继发了急性肾小球肾炎。

急性肾小球肾炎，又称急性肾炎，可发生于任何年龄段，尤其多发于 5～15 岁的儿童及青少年。它多于急性链球菌感染两周后急性起病。近年来，由于抗生素普遍使用等原因，其发病率已呈下降趋势。

在临床症状上，约有80%的患者可出现晨起颜面部的水肿，约有30%的患者可出现肉眼血尿，部分患者可出现轻、中度蛋白尿或一过性高血压，少数重症患者甚至出现充血性心力衰竭。

在临床诊断上，链球菌感染后1~3周发生急性肾炎综合征，伴血清C3一过性降低，可考虑临床诊断。必要时可进行肾穿刺活检明确诊断。

在临床治疗上，以支持与对症治疗为主，包括卧床休息、限盐、降压、利尿消肿等，有感染时可抗感染治疗。急性肾炎属自限性疾病，多数预后良好，但仍有少数患者病情恶化或转为"慢性"。中医药早期干预对减轻患者水肿、尿血、咽痛症状，改善临床预后具有积极作用。

中医观察到大部分急性肾炎患者，会很快出现颜面部及双下肢水肿，所以将其归属于"水肿"范畴，并用"阳水水肿"来形容水肿发病迅速。在病因病机上，认为其发病多与外感风邪或疮毒内犯有关。

中医在临床治疗上，常采用疏风、清热、宣肺、解毒、利水等祛邪的治法，常用越婢加术汤、麻黄连翘赤小豆汤等中医经典方剂。

越婢加术汤是汉代医圣张仲景创制的经典名方，由麻黄、生石膏、白术、生姜、大枣、甘草组成，可以疏风清热、宣肺行水。当急性肾炎水肿发展特别迅速，颜面部水肿继而四肢全身都肿，尤其是伴有发热、恶寒、肢体酸楚、咽喉肿痛等感冒症状时，使用越婢加术汤最为合适。

麻黄连翘赤小豆汤也是由医圣张仲景创制，由麻黄、连翘、赤小豆、杏仁、生梓白皮、生姜、大枣、甘草组成，可以宣肺解毒、利湿消肿。本方适用于皮肤感染性疾病如脓疱疮后继发的急性肾炎水肿。当患者水肿起病急，并伴有皮肤疮疡、小便量少且颜色发红、怕风、发热、舌质红、苔薄黄、脉浮数时，就可以使用这个方剂进行治疗。

当急性肾炎迁延不愈，转为"慢性"时，水肿可能迟迟不消退。中医学把这种缠绵不愈的水肿称为"阴水水肿"。在治疗上，常采用健脾、补肾、温阳、利水等补益为主的治法，常选用实脾饮、真武汤、金匮肾气丸等中医经典方剂，具有一定疗效。

2. IgA肾病

IgA肾病是目前世界范围内最常见的原发性肾小球疾病，在欧洲和亚洲占原发性肾小球疾病的 15% ~ 40%，它也是终末期肾病的重要病因。IgA 肾病可发生于任何年龄段，尤其多见于 20 ~ 30 岁男性。

在临床表现上，IgA 肾病起病隐匿，常表现为无症状性血尿或伴蛋白尿，一些患者可表现为高血压、肾病综合征和不同程度的肾功能损害。

在临床诊断上，若发现与上呼吸道感染相关的镜下血尿和蛋白尿，应考虑 IgA 肾病，必要时应行肾活检免疫病理检查以明确诊断。

在临床治疗上，对仅表现为单纯镜下血尿的患者，无须治疗，但需定期复查；对感染后反复发作性肉眼血尿患者，应积极使用无肾毒性药物抗感染；对蛋白尿或高血压伴蛋白尿患者，可使用 ARB/ACEI 控制尿蛋白及血压，以保护肾功能，延缓疾病进展。

IgA 肾病预后并不乐观，10 年肾脏存活率在 80% 左右，20 年在 65% 左右，部分患者治疗效果不佳，甚至快速进展为肾衰竭。研究发现，中医药的及时干预治疗，对于缓解不适症状、改善血尿及蛋白尿、延缓肾功能恶化有一定作用。

在中医学中，IgA 肾病属于"肾风""水肿"等范畴。在病因上多与外感邪气，正气虚弱有关。在病机上，邪犯咽喉，人体正气不足，不能御邪，邪气深入侵袭肾脏从而发病。

在临床治疗上，经典名方防己黄芪汤和中成药黄葵胶囊在临床运用非常广泛。防己黄芪汤出自汉代医圣张仲景的著作《金匮要略》，本方由防己、黄芪、白术、甘草、生姜、大枣组成，具有益气祛风、健脾利水功效。临床上常用来治疗伴随有容易汗出、怕风，容易出现眼睑或下肢水肿、肢体关节疼痛的 IgA 肾病。现代研究发现，该方可以减轻肾小球系膜细胞的炎症反应，减少系膜细胞增殖和系膜外基质的沉积，从而延缓 IgA 肾病进展。

黄葵胶囊是我国研制的治疗 IgA 肾病等慢性肾病的中成药，尤其适合于有浮肿、腰痛、蛋白尿、血尿和舌苔黄腻等湿热证表现的慢性肾病患者。黄葵胶囊的主要成分为黄蜀葵花，这是一种我国传统药用植物。据《本草纲目》记载，黄蜀葵花具有清热利湿、解毒消肿功效。黄葵胶囊自上市以来，有超过 15000 例慢性肾脏病患者参与了相关的临床研究，其疗效与安全性获得了广大临床医生的认可。中国工程院陈香美院士牵头开展了黄葵胶囊治疗原发性肾小球疾病有效性及安全性的随机对照双盲多中心临床试验，共纳入 414 例原发性肾小球疾病患者，研究发现，与氯沙坦相比，黄葵胶囊干预 24 周后，24h 尿蛋白下降率显著优于氯沙坦，且未发生严重不良反应。该项成果发表在 *American Journal of Kidney Diseases* 上，是肾病中成药高级别循证医学证据。

黄葵胶囊内容物为棕褐色粉末，味微甘、苦，服用方法是每次 5 粒，每日 3 次，8 周为一个疗程。

参考文献

ZHANG L, LI P, XING C Y, et al. Efficacy and safety of Abelmoschus manihot for primary glomerular disease: a prospective, multicenter randomized controlled clinical trial[J]. Am J Kidney Dis, 2014, 64 (1): 57-65.

3. 慢性肾衰竭

大家可能听过一些人因为慢性肾衰竭需要"透析"或"换肾"，但却不太了解什么是慢性肾衰竭。慢性肾衰竭是世界各国都面临的重大公共卫生问题，它是各种慢性肾脏病进展到后期的共同结局。目前国际上把慢性肾脏病分为 5 期，慢性肾衰竭则代表慢性肾脏病中肾小球滤过率下降至失代偿期的部分，主要为第 4～5 期。

在病因上，导致慢性肾衰竭的主要病因包括糖尿病肾病、高血压肾小动脉硬化、原发性或继发性肾小球疾病等。高血压、高血糖、高血脂、蛋白尿、低蛋白血症及吸烟、使用肾毒性药物等都是慢性肾脏病进展为慢性肾衰竭的重要危险因素。

在临床症状上，慢性肾衰竭常表现为水肿、乏力、腰酸、夜尿增多等。此外，当累及心血管、呼吸、消化等系统时，还会表现为喘憋、气短、恶心、呕吐等不适。

在临床诊断上，主要依据病史、临床表现及肾功能检查进行诊断。

在临床治疗上，包括控制血压、血糖、蛋白尿，纠正酸中毒和水、电解质紊乱，纠正贫血、低钙血症、高脂血症及预防感染等并发症，以及透析治疗。在临床治疗中发现，部分患者在慢性肾功能不全时即选择中西医结合治疗，有利于改善症状，保护肾功能，延缓终末期肾病的发生。

在中医学中，慢性肾衰竭属于"关格"范畴。在病因上，多与阴阳气血亏虚，血瘀、痰浊、水毒内停有关。在病机上，则为正虚御邪不能，邪毒侵袭肾脏，肾络瘀阻，水道不利，气化失司，久则发为肾衰竭。

在临床治疗上，大黄、黄芪等单味中药对慢性肾衰竭的治疗作用逐渐被阐明，由大黄、黄芪等组成的中成药尿毒清颗粒因其可靠的疗效和安全性，在慢性肾衰竭中得到广泛运用。

　　大黄为蓼科植物掌叶大黄、唐古特大黄或药用大黄的干燥根及根茎。大黄味苦、性寒，归脾、胃、大肠、肝、心包经，具有泻下攻积、清热解毒、利湿退黄等功效。现代药理学研究发现，大黄中的大黄酸等有效成分能抑制肾间质纤维化和肾小球纤维化及硬化，保护组织细胞，改善微循环和肾功能。黄芪为豆科植物蒙古黄芪或膜荚黄芪的干燥根。黄芪味甘、性微温，归脾、肺经，具有利水消肿、托毒生肌、补气升阳、益气固表等功效。黄芪中的活性成分黄芪甲苷等成分可以改善肾脏微循环，对慢性肾衰竭肾脏具有抗纤维化及潜在的抗炎作用。

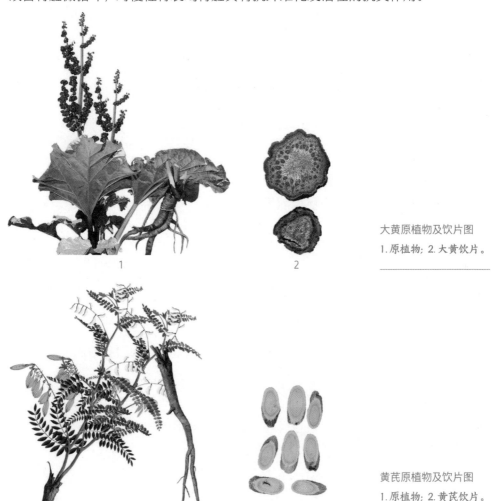

大黄原植物及饮片图
1.原植物; 2.大黄饮片。

黄芪原植物及饮片图
1.原植物; 2.黄芪饮片。

　　尿毒清颗粒由大黄、黄芪、甘草、茯苓、白术、何首乌、川芎、菊花、丹参、半夏等中药组成，具有通腑降浊、健脾利湿、活血化瘀功效。针对慢性肾衰竭患者，该药不仅可以降低肌酐、尿素氮水平，改善肾功能，而且可以改善慢性肾衰竭导致的贫血、低血钙、高血脂，现已入选我国《中成药治疗优势病种临床应用指南》，为治疗慢性肾衰竭的"强推荐"中成药。中成药尿毒清颗粒剂量规格为每袋 5g，服用方法为温开水冲服。值得注意的是，其服法特殊，要求患者每日服用 4 次，在 6 时、12 时、18 时各服一袋，22 时服用两袋。

除了内服药物，在中医治疗上，也可运用针刺、艾灸、穴位贴敷、中药灌肠等手段，对慢性肾衰竭进行综合干预，对于减轻患者水肿等症状及改善生活质量具有一定作用。

4. 尿路感染

不少人都体会过尿频、尿急、尿痛等不适，有的人甚至还伴有发热、寒战、腰痛等症状，这多半是尿路感染引起的。尿路感染是病原微生物在尿路中生长繁殖而引起的一种常见感染性疾病，全球每年约有 1.3 亿 ~ 1.75 亿人患此病。

在病因上，本病与细菌、真菌、支原体等病原体有关。其中，最常见的病原体是以大肠埃希菌为代表的革兰氏阴性杆菌，占单纯性尿路感染的75% ~ 90%。

在临床表现上，患者常出现以尿频、尿急、尿痛为主的膀胱刺激征，有的还会出现排尿困难、尿液混浊等。若是发生了急性肾盂肾炎，还可能会出现发热、寒战、头痛和腰痛。

在临床诊断上，除了依据尿路感染的临床表现，还应进行尿常规、细菌涂片和细菌培养来明确致病菌。

随着诊查手段的进步和抗生素的广泛使用，大部分尿路感染患者在积极、合理的抗感染治疗后可完全康复。但也有部分患者，由于泌尿系结构异常或免疫力低下等原因，感染始终无法得到良好控制而反复发作，单用西药控制不理想，所以希望联合中药治疗，减少发作频次。

在中医学中，尿路感染属于"淋证"范畴，病位在肾与膀胱，在病因上，与体虚劳倦、外感湿热毒邪有关。在病机上，与湿热蕴结下焦，肾与膀胱气化不利有关。

在临床治疗上，常用当归贝母苦参丸、八正散等中医经典方剂及三金片等中成药。当归贝母苦参丸出自汉代医圣张仲景的著作《金匮要略》。该方由当归、贝母、苦参 3 味中药以相同的比例研磨成粉，再用蜂蜜调和做成药丸，具有清热利尿，养血安胎的作用。从原书记载可以得知，医圣张仲景用此方来治疗妊娠期尿路感染。在现代临床运用中，只要尿路感染出现小便涩痛、尿黄、大便干以及色红苔黄腻、脉滑数这类湿热征象，都可以灵活运用此方进行治疗。

八正散记载于宋代《太平惠民和剂局方》，由车前子、瞿麦、萹蓄、滑石、栀子、甘草、木通、大黄8味中药组成，是自古以来治疗尿路感染的名方，具有清热解毒、利湿通淋的功效。八正散适合于尿频、尿急、尿痛症状突出，并伴有尿液混浊、小腹急痛、口渴、舌红苔黄腻、脉滑数的急性尿路感染患者。以八正散为基本方研制的中成药八正合剂，已在临床上投入使用，其规格为每瓶150ml或200ml，服用方法为每次口服15～20ml，每日3次。

三金片具有清热解毒、利湿通淋的功效，是治疗尿路感染的常用中成药。它主要由金樱根、菝葜、羊开口、金沙藤、积雪草等中药组成，特别适合具有尿频、尿急、尿痛、小便短赤、烦热、口苦、舌红苔黄腻、脉滑数等明显下焦湿热表现的尿路感染患者。一项纳入8项随机对照试验，共包括790名尿路感染的荟萃分析研究发现，三金片与左氧氟沙星等抗生素疗效相当，三金片与抗生素合用可以提高治愈率、总有效率和细菌清除率，并降低感染复发率。三金片分为2种规格，小片每片重0.18g，大片每片重0.29g，服用方法为口服，小片每次5片，大片每次3片，均为一日3～4次。

参考文献

LYU J, XIE Y, SUN M, et al. Sanjin tablet combined with antibiotics for treating patients with acute lower urinary tract infections: a meta-analysis and GRADE evidence profile[J]. Exp Ther Med, 2020, 19(1): 683-695.

5. 尿失禁

尿失禁是指储尿期膀胱内压力超过尿道阻力而出现尿液从尿道外口溢出的现象，就是大家所说的"憋不住尿"，常被戏称为"成年人的崩溃"。对于患者而言，这却是一件非常令人尴尬的事，常严重影响到他们的身心健康与社会交往。然而，这种羞于启齿的疾病，居然困扰到全球近20亿人。尿失禁在女性中的发病率明显高于男性，在我国，女性群体中约有三分之一的人受此困扰，7%左右的人有明显的尿失禁表现。

在临床表现上，患者主要表现为在咳嗽、喷嚏、大笑、运动或搬运重物时，或者尿急还来不及赶到厕所时，甚至在喝水、听到流水声、情绪紧张时，尿液便不受控制地流出。一些患者有时还会伴随尿血、排尿困难或盆腔疼痛等症状。

在临床诊断上，一般依据上述典型临床表现，结合相关产科、妇科病史和体格检查便可以诊断。

在临床治疗上，可以进行以凯格尔运动为代表的盆底肌训练，来改善盆底功能，提高尿道稳定性。也可以使用度洛西汀、雌激素等药物治疗，或尿道中段吊带术等手术治疗。不少患者为避免手术治疗带来的创伤，常更倾向于选择药物治疗、康复训练等非手术治疗方式。

在中医学中，尿失禁属于"遗溺""小便不禁"范畴，病位在膀胱与肾，病因上与久病体虚、胎产过多等相关。在病机上，则是由于体虚劳倦、胎产过多损耗肾气，肾气不固则膀胱失约，所以出现小便不受控制。

在临床治疗上，常选用以金匮肾气丸为代表的中医经典名方以及针刺进行治疗。金匮肾气丸是汉代医圣张仲景创制的经典名方，由桂枝、附子、生地黄、山药、山茱萸、泽泻、茯苓、牡丹皮8味中药组成，是温补肾阳的代表方。该方可温煦肾阳、填补肾精，使肾气充足、膀胱开阖有度，特别适合伴有腰膝酸软、怕冷、四肢发凉及舌色淡、脉沉弱的尿失禁患者。该方已被制成中成药投入市场，一般每瓶360丸，服用方法为每次吃25丸，一天2次，但需注意孕妇忌服。

以针刺为代表的中医治疗方式，在治疗女性尿失禁方面同样显示出独特的临床优势，已在临床广泛运用。2017年，国际顶级医学杂志《美国医学会杂志》（*The Journal of the American Medical Association*，JAMA）发表了由中国中医科学院刘保延教授和广安门医院刘志顺主任医师团队完成的"电针对女性压力性尿失禁漏尿量疗效的随机临床试验"研究报告。研究发现，给予电针针刺腰骶部中髎穴、会阳穴，每周3次，疗程共6周，可

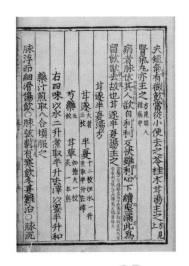

肾气丸条文

有效缓解女性压力性尿失禁，且疗效持久、很少出现不良反应，为广大尿失禁患者带来了福音。

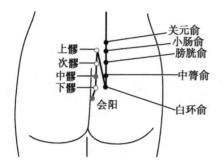

中髎穴、会阳穴

参考文献

LIU Z S, LIU Y, XU H F, et al. Effect of electroacupuncture on urinary leakage among women with stress urinary incontinence: a randomized clinical trial[J]. JAMA, 2017, 317 (24): 2493-2501.

第五节
血液系统疾病

一、血液系统疾病概述

血液系统疾病是原发于造血系统的疾病或者影响造血系统伴血液异常改变的疾病。造血系统由血液、骨髓、单核-巨噬细胞系统和淋巴组织四部分组成。凡是涉及造血系统病理生理，并且以之为主要表现的疾病，均属于血液病范畴。临床常见的血液系统疾病包括贫血、白细胞减少症和粒细胞缺乏症、脾功能亢进、白血病、血友病、紫癜等。

在临床治疗上，主要包括放化疗、造血干细胞及骨髓移植、脾切除术等。然而，基于血液的特殊性，大多数血液病具有病程长，并发症多，容易复发，控制率低等问题。感染、出血、凝血功能障碍，脾切除后血小板增多、免疫系统功能下降及血栓等后遗症等严重影响患者生活质量。

在中医学中，血液系统疾病属于"虚劳"等范畴。近年来，随着砷剂治疗白血病的临床证据在 *New England Journal of Medicine* 上发表后，中医药治疗血液病的优势逐渐得到全球关注。除砷剂之外，大菟丝子饮治疗再生障碍性贫血，青黄散治疗慢性粒细胞白血病及骨髓增生异常综合征，复方黄黛片治疗急性早幼粒细胞白血病等的大量临床证据得以逐步揭晓。在本节中，将围绕贫血、再生障碍性贫血、白细胞减少、白血病 4 种血液病，重点介绍中医药临床诊疗优势与方案。

二、血液系统疾病各论

1. 贫血

在日常生活中，常会有人觉得自己浑身乏力，面色苍白，气色不好，尤其是女性。身边人大多会说一句：你是不是贫血了？可见贫血在人群中发病率不低。下面我们就来深入了解一下这种我们看似熟悉疾病。

贫血是指单位容积血液内红细胞数和血红蛋白含量低于正常。根据血红蛋白数量可以诊断贫血。对于男性，血红蛋白低于 120g/L 就可以诊断贫血，对于女性血红蛋白低于 110g/L，才可诊断贫血。根据血红蛋白的数量，贫血一般可分为轻度、中度和重度。血红蛋白在 90～110/120g/L 时，可以诊断为轻度贫血；血红蛋白在 60～90g/L 时，可诊断为中度贫血；血红蛋白低于 60g/L 时，可诊断为重度贫血。

造成贫血的原因有很多，包括缺铁、出血、溶血、造血功能障碍等。在临床症状上，表现为头晕，乏力，失眠，多梦，记忆力减退，皮肤、眼睑苍白等症状，主要以皮肤、指甲、眼睑苍白为主要辨别特征。在贫血中，缺铁性贫血最常见。

在临床治疗上，主要包括输血的对症治疗和补充铁剂、叶酸等对因治疗。然而，在临床上，患者常因头晕反复发作，症状缓解不明显，进而求助于中医药治疗。

在中医中，贫血属于"血虚""虚劳"等范畴。在病机上，贫血属于虚证，以脾气虚弱，肾虚髓亏为主。中医学认为，脾胃为气血生化之源，血的生成与脾的关系最为密切。饮食不节、劳倦过度、久病体虚等皆可损及脾胃功能，导致贫血。在临床中，经典名方当归补血汤与归脾汤最为常用。

当归补血汤出自金元时期的著名医家李东垣的《内外伤辨惑论》，由补气的黄芪和补血的当归按5：1的比例组成。处方中既用黄芪补脾肺之气，又有当归养血补血，尤其适用于气血亏虚的贫血患者。这类患者可表现为头晕目眩，动则倦怠乏力，心悸，气短，舌淡嫩，苔薄白，脉沉弱。在古代，还以当归补血汤为基础方，加减化裁出很多益气补血的良方。圣愈汤就是一个例子，由黄芪、人参、当归、地黄、白芍、川芎组成，能够治疗失血兼有贫血患者。

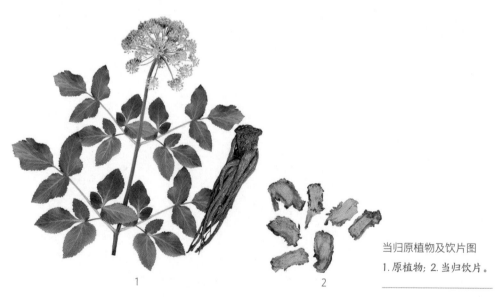

当归原植物及饮片图
1.原植物；2.当归饮片。

归脾汤出自《济生方》，由人参、白术、茯苓、黄芪、炙甘草、当归、远志、酸枣仁、龙眼肉、木香、大枣组成。本方有益气养血，健脾补心的功效，尤其适用于心脾血虚证患者，临床表现为面色萎黄，倦怠，神疲，自汗，心悸，气短，头晕目眩，食欲不振，恶心呕吐，腹痛腹泻，舌淡胖，脉细弱。现代药理学研究发现，本方有增强造血功能作用。现今临床常用的中成药归脾丸就出自于归脾汤原方，服用方法为每次 9g，每日 3 次。

2. 再生障碍性贫血

再生障碍性贫血为一种骨髓衰竭综合征，简单来说就是骨髓造血功能下降。我国再生障碍性贫血年发病率为 0.74/10 万。患者全血细胞减少，临床表现为贫血，或合并有感染和出血。本病发病以青壮年居多，男性多于女性。

在病因上，获得性再生障碍性贫血目前病因不明确，苯及其衍生物的职业暴露是最为明确的病因。其他如抗肿瘤药物、电离辐射、病毒感染等也有报道。

在临床症状上，重型再生障碍性贫血起病急，发展迅速，以出血、感染和发热为首发症状。本病预后差，死亡率高。非重型再生障碍性贫血起病和发展缓慢，以乏力、心悸、面色苍白等贫血表现为主。

在临床治疗上，西医学常以免疫抑制剂、骨髓移植、雄激素刺激骨髓造血，以及其他支持疗法如控制感染、成分输血等为主要治疗手段。然而，免疫抑制剂可能引起免疫系统功能下降，易合并感染，有一定的肝肾毒性；骨髓移植适用人群范围狭窄；雄激素治疗存在一定程度的雄性化现象和肝毒性等。很多再生障碍性贫血患者会寻求中医药的积极治疗。中医在慢性再生障碍性贫血的治疗中具有一定优势，可减少并发症，如感染、皮肤瘀点、牙龈出血等，调节免疫系统功能，减轻西药不良反应，提高患者生活质量。

在中医学中，再生障碍性贫血属于"急劳""髓劳""虚劳"等范畴。在病因上，本病多由邪毒直中伤髓所致，邪毒即包括药物、辐射等。在病机上，本病以髓亏精虚为本，气血不足为标。

在临床上，常用经典名方炙甘草汤和中药注射剂黄芪注射液。炙甘草汤出自《伤寒论》，由炙甘草、人参、干姜、桂枝、麦冬、生地黄、火麻仁、阿胶、大枣组成，具有益气复脉，滋阴通阳的作用。因炙甘草汤能够有效提高血细胞数量，常用于治疗各类由出血、失血或其他原因导致的血细胞减少，如再生障碍性贫血、重度贫血、血小板减少及白细胞减少等。现代药理学研究表明，方中人参、阿胶均能提升骨髓造血功能，君药炙甘草，生地黄均能提高机体免疫力外，生地黄还有部分抵抗电离辐射的作用。

黄芪注射液，由单味中药黄芪加辅料碳酸氢钠等精制而成，具有益气固表，健脾补中，扶正祛邪的功效。药理学研究表明黄芪具有明显的刺激骨髓造血的作用，还可以双向调节免疫反应，增强机体抵抗力，能够减少感染等并发症的发生。临床一般肌内注射，一次 2~4ml，一日 1~2 次，或静脉滴注，一次 10~20ml，一日 1 次。

参考文献

熊兴江. 基于现代病理生理及 CCU 急危重症病例的炙甘草汤方证溯源及其复律，转窦，止血，升血小板，补虚临床运用 [J]. 中国中药杂志，2019，44（18）：19.

3. 白细胞减少

白细胞减少症是指周围血白细胞持续低于 4×10^9/L。白细胞成分中一半以上为中性粒细胞，若周围血中性粒细胞低于 2×10^9/L，则称为粒细胞减少。

在病因上，白细胞减少与肿瘤放、化疗直接杀伤外周白细胞，各类药物如解热镇痛药布洛芬、阿司匹林等，抗甲状腺药，抗生素，心血管药物等，感染及免疫系统疾病，以及理化因素，包括电离辐射及苯、甲苯等密切相关。

在临床症状上，本病多为慢性过程，可伴有头晕、乏力、食欲减退、低热、腰痛等表现，若其中粒细胞少于 1×10^9/L，可出现口腔炎、中耳炎、支气管炎、肺炎、肾盂肾炎等继发感染。

在临床治疗上，包括去除病因，劳逸结合，适当锻炼，控制感染，使用糖皮质激素及促进粒细胞生成药物。由于部分患者不耐受糖皮质激素等治疗的不良反应，且部分对症治疗存在容易复发的缺点，不能有效改善白细胞减少患者的生活质量，因此在临床上，很多患者积极寻求中医药治疗。

在中医学中，本病属于"虚损""虚劳"范畴。在病因上，多与感受外邪、药毒，禀赋不足，饮食失调，劳倦内伤，久病、大病有关。在病机上，本病为本虚标实之症，多属气血亏虚、脾肾两虚。

在临床上，常用经典名方八珍汤和中成药地榆升白片。八珍汤出自《正体类要》，由人参、白术、茯苓、甘草、当归、熟地黄、芍药、川芎组成，内含健脾益气的四君子汤和养血补血的四物汤，是气血并补的经典方剂。临床上广泛应用于白细胞减少伴见气短懒言、四肢倦怠、食欲减退等虚弱性症状。现代药理学研究证实，八珍汤具有提高免疫力、促进造血功能的作用，还有一定的杀伤肿瘤细胞作用。临床研究也发现，本方不仅能用于改善由肿瘤、放化疗、甲巯咪唑等各种原因导致的白细胞减少，还能有效改善相关临床症状，提高生活质量。

地榆升白片主要成分为中药地榆。与利血生、重组人粒细胞刺激因子等这一类昂贵药品相比，其具有疗效稳定且价格低廉、安全性高的优点。目前已被广泛运用于肿瘤放化疗后，服用抗甲状腺药甲巯咪唑、干扰素等导致的白细胞减少。现代药理学研究表明地榆具有促进骨髓细胞增殖，增加骨髓有核细胞数量，增加外周血白细胞、红细胞、血小板数量的作用，并能有效止血。其临床服用方法为口服，每次2~4片，每日3次。

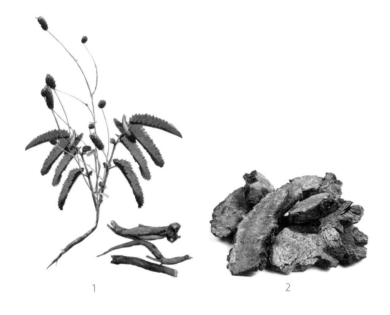

地榆原植物及饮片图
1. 原植物；2. 地榆饮片。

4. 白血病

白血病，俗称"血癌"，是一种造血干细胞恶性克隆性疾病，属于恶性肿瘤。在我国，白血病年发病率有逐年升高趋势。

在发病原因上，本病与病毒感染、电离辐射、化学物质、遗传等有关。其中，某些抗肿瘤药物与本病密切相关。流行病学调查发现，苯及其衍生物、染料、染发剂的长期职业暴露或生活接触为重要原因。

在临床症状上，急性白血病发病急骤，常伴见高热、感染、出血、贫血、肝脾肿大、骨骼肌关节疼痛、恶心呕吐等表现。实验室检查中贫血及血小板减少最为常见，骨髓象增生明显活跃或极度活跃为其诊断的主要依据。慢性白血病常以肝脾肿大为主，也可见低热、出汗和消瘦等临床表现。

在临床治疗上，需要结合临床分型和预后分层制订有效的治疗方案，目前主要包括化疗、放疗、靶向治疗、免疫治疗、干细胞移植等。虽然化疗为目前临床主要治疗手段，但其副作用大，临床易复发，且治疗费用较高，给患者带来了沉重的医疗负担。

在中医学中，白血病属于"虚劳""热劳""百日劳""癥积"等范畴。在病机上，本病存在热毒、痰凝、血瘀、正虚，且互为因果，形成虚实夹杂之证。近年来，中医药治疗白血病的靶向抗癌、改善症状、毒副作用少、中西药联用减毒增效等临床优势逐渐受到关注，尤其是三氧化二砷治疗白血病取得突破性进展。

癌灵1号注射液，由中药砒霜研制而成，主要成分为三氧化二砷和亚砷酸。研究表明，其对急性早幼粒细胞白血病安全缓解率达91%，慢性粒细胞白血病总缓解率为72%，对淋巴瘤总缓解率为70%。由于其能透过血–脑屏障，故在治疗中很大程度避免了合并中枢神经系统白血病的发生。临床观察未见强烈毒性反应和骨髓抑制现象，部分患者会有恶心、胃胀、皮肤瘙痒等反应，停药或对症治疗后可消失。此外，癌灵1号注射液还能促进巨核细胞增殖，促进血小板生成。砷剂治疗主要机制是诱导白血病细胞分化、凋亡，不同于以往的放化疗是无选择性的，不分好坏细胞全部杀死。此药选择性地针对白血病细胞而对正常细胞绕路而行，所以疗效更加确切，安全性也更高。在癌灵1号注射液基础上，国内相继开展了砷剂治疗白血病的临床与基础研究，并很快受到国际关注。Sloan-Ketting 等人对 12 例急性早幼粒细胞白血病常规治疗后复发患者给予砷剂治疗，11 例得到完全缓解。该研究于《新英格兰医学杂志》（*The New England Journal of Medicine*）发表后，国际上开始普遍接受砷剂治疗白血病的临床疗效。

参考文献

SOIGNET S L, MASLAK P, WANG Z G, et al. Complete remission after treatment of acute promyelocytic leukemia with arsenic trioxide[J]. New England Journal of Medicine, 1998, 339 (19): 1341-1348.

第六节
内分泌与代谢疾病

一、内分泌与代谢疾病概述

我们经常会见到有的人一旦出现长痤疮、月经不调、怕热多汗、失眠等症状，或者体检时发现血糖、血脂升高或激素水平异常，就会怀疑自己是不是"内分泌失调了""代谢紊乱了"？其实，这样的疑虑不无道理。

内分泌系统由垂体、甲状腺、肾上腺等内分泌腺和分布在身体各处的内分泌组织和细胞构成，各种激素由其产生并分泌入血，作用于靶器官及靶组织，维持人体的正常生理功能。内分泌与代谢性疾病种类非常多，最常见的包括甲状腺功能亢进、甲状腺功能减退、甲状腺结节等甲状腺疾病，糖尿病以及高脂血症等疾病。

在临床治疗上，对于功能亢进患者，可以选择手术切除、药物治疗等方式来减少内分泌肿瘤或增生组织释放激素；对于功能减退的患者，可补充相应的外源激素，如甲状腺功能减退者予以补充左甲状腺素钠。然而，我们发现，部分患者不满足于长期口服药物维持，包括长期口服左甲状腺素、降糖药、降脂药等，部分患者还因西药治疗后的不良反应，进而寄希望于中医药治疗。

近年来，中医药在内分泌与代谢性疾病的临床治疗上不断取得进展，并且越来越得到国际认可。内分泌与代谢性疾病属于中医"虚劳""瘿病""消渴""血浊"等疾病范畴。临床上发现，中医药在改善甲状腺功能、缩小甲状腺结节、调节糖脂代谢、减轻糖尿病并发症及改善相关临床症状方面，均显示出一定临床价值。本节将重点介绍中医药治疗甲状腺功能减退、甲状腺结节、血脂异常、糖尿病及其并发症的临床诊治方案。

二、内分泌与代谢疾病各论

1. 甲状腺功能减退症

甲状腺功能减退症，俗称"甲减"，是指由各种原因导致血中甲状腺激素水平降低，或甲状腺激素抵抗，而表现出的一种低代谢综合征。在病因上常与自身免疫性甲状腺炎、甲状腺手术损伤及 ^{131}I 治疗等相关。

在临床表现上，早期或轻症患者可能不会有特异性症状，而典型患者可能会出现畏寒、乏力、嗜睡、记忆减退、反应迟钝、少汗、月经紊乱、体重增加、水肿等人体代谢功能减退和交感神经活性减低症状。

在临床诊断上，应询问甲状腺相关病史如手术史、^{131}I 治疗史，结合患者临床表现，并进行血清 TSH、TT_4、FT_4 检查。

在临床治疗上，目前主要的治疗方式为左甲状腺素治疗，常用药物就是大家所熟知的"优甲乐"，治疗目标是把血清 TSH 和甲状腺激素稳定在正常水平。服药效果较好，但要求患者终身规律服药，并定期复查激素指标，在一定程度上，存在诸多不便。中医药在治疗甲状腺功能减退症方面具有一定的临床价值与意义，对于改善甲状腺功能减退相关症状具有一定的优势。

在中医学中，甲状腺功能减退症属于"虚劳""水肿""瘿劳"范畴。在病因上，与情志内伤、体虚劳倦、饮食水土及体质因素密切相关。在病机上，由于情志内伤、久病体虚等各种因素导致脏腑功能减退，进而出现一系列以"虚耗"为主的表现。甲状腺功能减退症最常见的症状包括畏寒、乏力、嗜睡、记忆减退、反应迟钝等全身低代谢、低交感神经兴奋性症状，就属于中医学"肾阳亏虚"范畴。

在临床治疗上，常选用经典名方金匮肾气丸与真武汤进行治疗。另外，也可选用艾灸、针刺等中医外治法。金匮肾气丸是汉代医圣张仲景创制的千古名方，由附子、桂枝、生地黄、山药、山茱萸、泽泻、茯苓、牡丹皮 8 味中药组成，具有温补肾阳功效。在临床上，可用于出现畏寒、精神不振、嗜睡、腰膝酸冷、水肿等肾阳亏虚证表现的甲状腺功能减退症患者的临床治疗。金匮肾气丸现在已经被研制成中成药，并在临床广泛运用。其规格一般为水蜜丸，每100 丸重 20g，每瓶 360 丸，用法用量为每次服 20 丸，一天 2 次，但需注意孕妇忌服。

真武汤也是医圣张仲景创制的经典名方，它由附子、茯苓、白术、白芍、生姜 5 味中药组成。它具有温阳利水的功效，适合属于脾肾阳虚，水湿内停证的甲状腺功能减退症患者。真武汤所治疗的甲状腺功能减退症患者，临床症状往往比肾气丸证患者严重，在畏寒肢冷、精神不振、反应迟钝等表现的基础上，往往还会出现水肿明显、舌胖大有齿痕、脉沉迟等水湿内停的表现。

针刺和艾灸也是中医治疗甲状腺功能减退症的方法。针刺或艾灸刺激肾俞穴、脾俞穴、关元穴、足三里穴等具有补益、强壮作用的穴位，对于缓解甲状腺功能减退症患者的畏寒、乏力、精神萎靡及水肿等症状具有一定疗效。

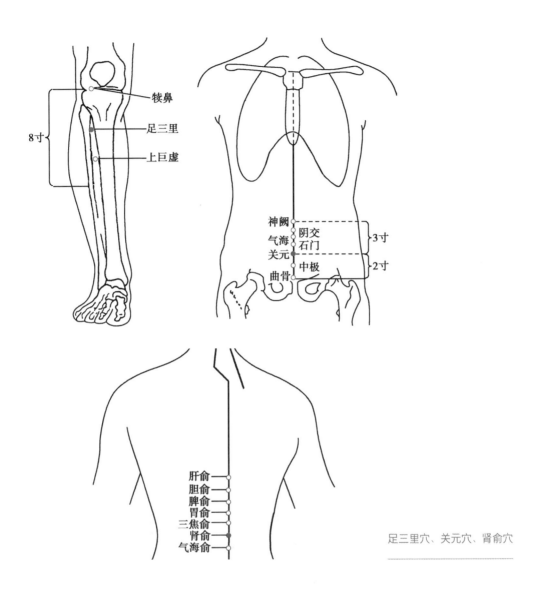

犊鼻

足三里

上巨虚

8寸

神阙
气海
关元
曲骨

阴交
石门

中极

3寸

2寸

肝俞
胆俞
脾俞
胃俞
三焦俞
肾俞
气海俞

足三里穴、关元穴、肾俞穴

2. 甲状腺结节

甲状腺结节在临床上极为常见，约有 50% 的人可在行超声检查时检出。大部分结节为良性腺瘤样结节或囊肿，但仍有 5% ~ 10% 的结节为恶性。许多人在体检发现甲状腺结节后，总是忧心忡忡，担心结节是恶性或者发生恶变。在病因上，其病因及发病机制目前仍不清楚。

在临床表现上，大多数甲状腺结节患者不会表现出任何临床症状。部分患者可因伴随甲状腺功能减退或甲状腺功能亢进而出现相应症状。一些恶性结节患者会由于肿块压迫气管而出现咳嗽、气促，压迫食管而出现吞咽困难等。

在临床诊断上，可结合既往病史、临床表现、血清 TSH 等实验室检查和超声检查综合判断。另外，超声引导下的细针抽吸细胞学检查是鉴别良恶性结节的金标准，准确度达 90% 以上，必要时可以选择。

在临床治疗上，恶性结节或结节出现压迫症状一般需要手术治疗，有自主分泌功能的结节可行放射性碘治疗。良性结节一般定期复查，不予特殊治疗。甲状腺结节由于其高发病率及恶变可能性，令许多患者心理压力极大。他们希望积极治疗，避免结节增大或恶变，进而寻求中医药治疗。

中医药对于缩小结节、改善体质等具有一定作用。在中医学中，甲状腺结节属于"瘿病""痰核"范畴。在病因上，多与情志内伤、饮食和水土不和及体质因素有关。在病机上，多与肝郁气滞，痰气瘀血搏结于颈前相关。

在临床治疗上，常用经典名方半夏厚朴汤与消瘰丸。半夏厚朴汤出自汉代医圣张仲景的《金匮要略》，由半夏、厚朴、茯苓、生姜、紫苏叶 5 味中药组成。该方主要是用来治疗"梅核气"，类似于慢性咽炎这类疾病。"异病同治"是中医学独特并且极具智慧的理论，意思是说不同疾病可以用相同的方法进行治疗，但前提是不同疾病具有相同或相似的病机。由于该方具有行气散结、降逆化痰的功效，契合甲状腺结节气滞、痰凝、血瘀的病机，所以现在也被广泛用来治疗甲状腺结节。需要注意的是，半夏厚朴汤的组成药物总体偏于温燥，容易耗伤人体阴液，并不适合咽干口燥、舌红苔黄、脉细数这类阴虚患者。

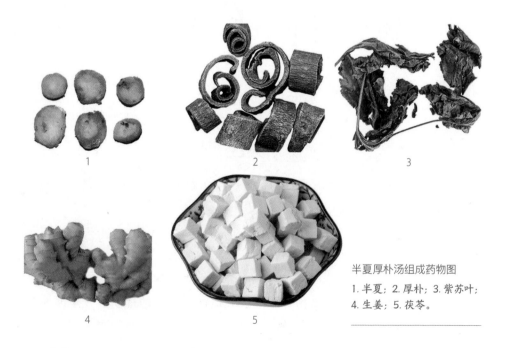

1 2 3

4 5

半夏厚朴汤组成药物图

1. 半夏；2. 厚朴；3. 紫苏叶；
4. 生姜；5. 茯苓。

消瘰丸记载于清代医家程国彭所著的《医学心悟》，由玄参、牡蛎、贝母3味中药组成，具有清热化痰、软坚散结的功效。与半夏厚朴汤不同，消瘰丸治疗的是肝郁化火、炼津为痰所致的结节，患者可伴有口苦、咽干、烦热、舌红苔黄或黄腻、脉弦数或滑数等痰热内蕴症状。内消瘰疬丸是在消瘰丸基础上研发的中成药，可以清热滋阴，消痰软坚，用以治疗甲状腺结节等疾病。

3. 血脂异常

我们在临床上经常看到，一些患有冠心病的老年人总是特别关心自己的血脂水平，担心血脂异常会加重冠状动脉病变，诱发心绞痛和心肌梗死。血脂异常一般是指血清中胆固醇、甘油三酯、低密度脂蛋白胆固醇水平升高，高密度脂蛋白胆固醇水平降低。我国成年人中血脂异常的比例高达40.4%，血脂异常是心脑血管疾病的重要危险因素。

在病因上，大多血脂异常是由遗传基因缺陷和环境因素综合作用导致，所以血脂异常有一定的家族聚集性。也有一些是由于甲状腺功能减退症、肾病综合征或服用某些药物引起。

在临床表现上，脂质沉积于血管内皮下会引起动脉粥样硬化，有的患者会因脂质局部沉积而出现"黄色瘤""角膜环"或眼底病变。

在临床诊断上，实验室血清检查可了解各脂质水平情况用以诊断。需注意的是，检查血脂前患者应禁食12小时以上，并且最后一餐应饮食清淡。

在临床治疗上，调脂首选他汀类药物，如常用的阿托伐他汀、瑞舒伐他汀等。当然，也需要进行合理饮食、减重、戒烟限酒或药物治疗等综合干预。

在中医学中，血脂异常属于"痰浊""血浊""逸病"等范畴。在病因上，多与脾肾亏虚、饮食肥甘、劳逸不当、痰浊阻滞及先天禀赋有关。在病机上，中医讲"身勤则强，逸则病"，现代人多过食肥甘厚味但缺乏锻炼，若加之先天禀赋不足，致使脾失健运、肾失气化，痰浊内生，流于血液，便会导致血脂异常。

在中医治疗上，中医经典名方葛根芩连汤和中成药血脂康胶囊常常被选用。葛根芩连汤出自汉代医圣张仲景的《伤寒论》，由葛根、黄芩、黄连、甘草4味中药组成，具有解表清里的作用。该方最初用来治疗感冒未康复，而邪气入里导致的腹泻。现代研究发现葛根芩连汤中葛根、黄连、黄芩均有较好的降血脂作用。该方尤其适合血脂异常伴口苦、烦渴、腹泻、舌红苔黄腻、脉滑数等症状的患者。

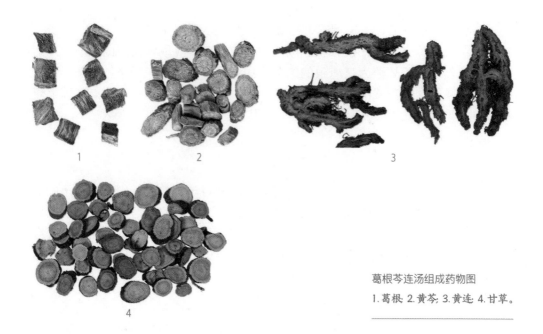

葛根芩连汤组成药物图

1.葛根 2.黄芩 3.黄连 4.甘草。

红曲是一种传统中药，为曲霉科真菌紫色红曲霉寄生在粳米上而成的红曲米，具有消食和胃、活血止痛和健脾的功效。血脂康胶囊是针对高脂血症研发出的一种调节血脂的中成药，它由接种特殊红曲菌的籼米制成，包含洛伐他汀等 13 种天然复合他汀以及不饱和脂肪酸、甾醇、黄酮类物质。血脂康胶囊具有化浊降脂、活血化瘀、健脾消食的功效，尤其适合有气短、乏力、头晕、胸闷、胸痛、腹胀、纳差等脾虚、痰阻、血瘀表现的血脂异常患者。由中国医学科学院阜外医院牵头开展的中国冠心病二级预防研究（CCSPS）是一项多中心随机双盲安慰剂对照临床试验，共纳入 4870 例有心肌梗死病史的冠心病患者，经过平均 3.5 年的治疗后发现，血脂康胶囊可使甘油三酯含量降低 13.2%，低密度脂蛋白胆固醇含量降低 20.2%，总胆固醇含量降低 15.0%，高密度脂蛋白胆固醇含量升高 4.9%。与安慰剂相比，血脂康可降低冠心病事件风险 45%、冠心病死亡风险 31%、全因死亡风险 33%。这一研究成果于 2008 年发表在《美国心脏病学杂志》上。该药已在临床上使用 20 余年，其疗效和安全性得到广泛认可。该药服用方法为每次口服 2 粒，一日 2 次。

参考文献

LU Z, KOU W, DU B, et al. Effect of Xuezhikang, an extract from red yeast Chinese rice, on coronary events in a Chinese population with previous myocardial infarction[J]. Am J Cardiol, 2008, 101 (12): 1689-1693.

4. 糖尿病前期

糖尿病前期是指已经出现空腹血糖受损、糖耐量异常，但还未达到糖尿病诊断标准的阶段。在我国，有超过三分之一的人处于糖尿病前期，如不干预，将有大量患者进展为糖尿病，给社会带来沉重的负担。

在临床表现上，大多患者不会出现特征性症状，仅在体检时发现空腹血糖、糖耐量试验或糖化血红蛋白异常。

在临床诊断上，当出现空腹血糖受损（FPG：5.6~6.9mmol/L）和糖耐量受损（OGTT2hPG：7.8~11.0mmol/L）时，或者糖化血红蛋白（HbA1c）5.7%~6.4%时，即可诊断。

在临床治疗上，主要包括合理饮食、加强锻炼等生活方式干预，也可服用二甲双胍等延缓病情进展。中医学认为，这种代谢异常的疾病与体质有很大关系。而在辨证调理体质，积极治疗糖尿病前期方面，中医药具有一定的疗效与优势。

在中医学中，糖尿病前期属于"消渴"等范畴。在病因上，与先天禀赋不足、饮食不节、劳倦内伤等相关。在病机上，以阴虚为本，燥热为标。

在临床治疗上，常用清代名医张锡纯创制的玉液汤以及中成药天芪降糖胶囊。玉液汤是降糖名方，由黄芪、天花粉、知母、葛根、五味子、山药、鸡内金7味中药组成。本方具有益气生津、固肾止渴功效，适用于伴有口渴、小便多、疲乏、脉虚无力等气阴两虚表现的糖尿病前期患者。现代药理学研究发现，方中的黄芪、天花粉、知母、葛根、五味子等中药，均有一定的降糖作用。

天芪降糖胶囊是在玉液汤基础上研制而成的中成药。它由天花粉、黄芪、女贞子、石斛、人参、地骨皮、黄连、山茱萸、墨旱莲、五味子10味中药组成，具有益气养阴、清热生津功效。该药适用于伴有倦怠乏力、口渴、五心烦热、自汗、盗汗、心悸、失眠、舌淡红、苔薄干、脉细弱或细数等气阴两虚症状的糖尿病前期患者。由中国中医科学院广安门医院仝小林院士牵头开展的一项纳入420例糖尿病前期患者的随机双盲多中心临床研究表明，与安慰剂相比，服用天芪降糖胶囊1年，可使糖尿病发生率降低32.1%。该药为硬胶囊，内容物为棕黄色至棕褐色粉末及颗粒，气微香，味苦。服用方法为每次口服5粒，一日3次。

参考文献

LIAN F, LI G, CHEN X, et al. Chinese herbal medicine Tianqi reduces progression from impaired glucose tolerance to diabetes: a double-blind, randomized, placebo-controlled, multicenter trial[J]. J Clin Endocrinol Metab, 2014, 99 (2): 648-655.

5. 糖尿病

糖尿病是一种在遗传和环境因素作用下，胰岛素分泌不足或利用缺陷引起糖代谢异常，以慢性高血糖为特征的代谢性疾病。在过去十年间，我国糖尿病患病人数从 9000 万增长至 1.4 亿。2021 年，全球糖尿病患病人数高达 5.37 亿，并且近年来发病率呈快速上升趋势，已成为全球重大公共卫生问题。

在临床表现上，糖尿病分为 1 型糖尿病和 2 型糖尿病，前者多于青少年时期发病，起病急而症状明显，后者一般为 40 岁以后发病，起病隐匿，一般症状较轻。无论是 1 型还是 2 型，可表现出典型的"三多一少"，即多饮、多食、多尿和体重减轻。此外，糖尿病常伴随各系统的并发症表现。当然，也有一些患者无明显症状，仅在体检或因病就医时偶然发现。

在临床诊断上，糖尿病的诊断常以"三多一少"、各种常见并发症临床表现以及糖尿病家族史等作为线索，基于空腹血浆葡萄糖（FPG）、随机血糖、糖化血红蛋白（HbA1c）、口服葡萄糖耐量试验（OGTT）2h 血糖（2hPG）值做出诊断。

在临床治疗上，糖尿病的治疗除生活方式干预外，常还包括促胰岛素分泌剂、胰岛素增敏剂、α-葡萄糖苷酶抑制剂、胰岛素、GLP-1 受体激动剂等。中医药对于控制高血糖、改善代谢紊乱、防治相关并发症具有一定的疗效与优势，因此不少患者会主动寻求中医药治疗。

在中医学中，糖尿病属于"消渴"范畴。在病因上，与先天禀赋不足、饮食不节、劳倦内伤等相关。在病机上，以阴虚为本，燥热为标，病久可能发生阴损及阳、阴阳俱虚。

在临床治疗上，常选用中医经典名方葛根芩连汤和中成药消渴丸。葛根芩连汤出自汉代医学著作《伤寒论》，由葛根、黄芩、黄连、甘草 4 味中药组成，具有解表清里的作用。该方最初用来治疗感冒未愈，邪气入里而导致的腹泻。现代临床研究发现，葛根芩连汤具有较好的降血糖作用，也广泛用于治疗糖尿病。本方尤其适合中医辨证为肠道湿热证的糖尿病患者，伴见口苦、烦渴、腹泻、舌红苔黄腻、脉滑数等症状。由中国中医科学院广安门医院仝小林院士开展的一项随机双盲对照临床试验，共纳入187例2型糖尿病患者，研究发现，与安慰剂组相比，葛根芩连汤干预12周，可显著改善空腹血糖和糖化血红蛋白水平，其作用机制与调节肠道微生物群有关。

消渴丸是以传统方剂玉泉丸和消渴方为基础，加入格列本脲制成的中西药复方制剂，包括黄芪、地黄、山药、葛根、天花粉、玉米须、五味子7味中药，具有滋肾养阴、益气生津的功效。它能有效降低糖尿病患者空腹血糖、口服葡萄糖耐量试验2h血糖及糖化血红蛋白水平。此外，由北京大学人民医院纪立农教授开展的一项随机对照双盲多中心临床试验，共纳入800例血糖控制不佳的2型糖尿病患者，研究发现，与格列本脲相比，消渴丸干预48周后可显著降低低血糖风险，且血糖也得以改善，提示消渴丸中的中药成分对格列本脲所致的低血糖有保护作用。消渴丸适合于中医辨证为气阴两虚证的糖尿病患者，临床表现为神疲、倦怠乏力、口渴、纳差、羸弱、舌淡红、苔薄白、脉虚或脉细无力。其规格为浓缩水丸，每瓶120丸，每10丸重2.5g。用法用量为每次口服5~10丸，一日2~3次。

参考文献

XU J, LIAN F, ZHAO L, et al. Structural modulation of gut microbiota during alleviation of type 2 diabetes with a Chinese herbal formula[J]. ISME J, 2015, 9 (3): 552-562.

JI L, TONG X, WANG H, et al. Efficacy and safety of traditional Chinese medicine for diabetes: a double-blind, randomised, controlled trial[J]. PLoS One, 2013, 8 (2): e56703. doi: 10.1371/journal. pone. 0056703.

6. 糖尿病并发症

在我国，有超过1/10的人患有糖尿病，每10个糖尿病患者中就有7个发生并发症。有人说，糖尿病不可怕，可怕的是糖尿病并发症，这其实是有一定道理的。糖尿病会造成眼、肾、血管、神经等组织器官的慢性进行性病变，导致多系统并发症的发生，甚至引起急性严重代谢紊乱。

在临床表现上，糖尿病可能引起急性严重代谢紊乱、各种慢性并发症，以及更容易并发感染性疾病。累及微血管时可能出现糖尿病肾病、糖尿病视网膜病变等，累及心脑肾动脉血管时可能出现冠心病、脑卒中、肾动脉硬化等。糖尿病足更是一种严重而可怕并且治疗费用高昂的并发症，常表现为足部难以愈合的溃疡和坏疽，不少患者甚至因此截肢。

在临床治疗上，根据不同的并发症，选择相应的治疗方案，包括补液、纠正电解质紊乱与酸碱失衡、胰岛素、抗感染、抗心衰等。尤其，在处理糖尿病足时，应积极抗感染、清创及换药。中医药在改善糖尿病并发症方面，具有一定疗效，现以糖尿病足为例介绍中医学的认识与治疗。

在中医学中，糖尿病足属于"消渴变证""脱疽"范畴。在病因病机上，糖尿病日久，阴阳俱损、血脉瘀滞、痰瘀热毒互结进而导致肉腐筋枯骨败。

在临床治疗上，常选用四妙勇安汤进行治疗。该方出自清代医书《验方新编》，由金银花、玄参、当归、甘草4味中药组成，具有清热解毒、活血止痛的功效，原书记载该方主治热毒炽盛的"脱疽"。临床常用于治疗如血栓闭塞性脉管炎、下肢深静脉栓塞以及糖尿病足等下肢疾病。现代药理学研究发现，金银花、玄参、当归、甘草都具有较好的抗感染、消炎、改善微循环等作用。需要注意的是，四妙勇安汤虽然药味少，但每味药用量却较大，量大是该方取效的关键。在实际运用时，可结合糖尿病足阴虚燥热、血败肉腐的基本病机，酌加具有滋阴清热降糖、托毒排脓生肌功效的中药。

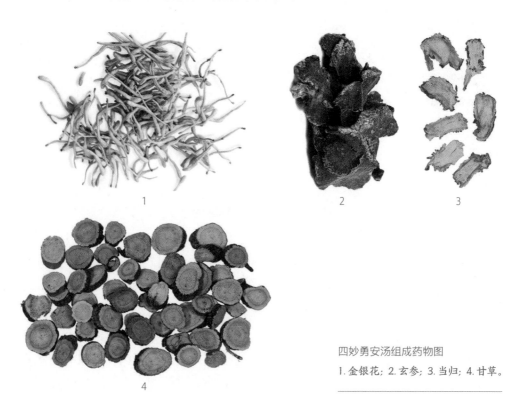

四妙勇安汤组成药物图

1.金银花；2.玄参；3.当归；4.甘草。

第七节
风湿性疾病

一、风湿性疾病概述

风湿性疾病是病因各不相同，但均累及到骨、关节及其周围组织的一组疾病。其病因多种多样，包括感染、免疫紊乱、内分泌紊乱、环境因素、遗传及退行性病变等。风湿性疾病发病率高，病程长，有一定的致残率，致死率不高。在临床症状上，关节和软组织疼痛是风湿性疾病最常见的症状之一，可出现关节僵硬、肿胀、变形、运动受限。

目前药物治疗是主要治疗手段，常用非甾体抗炎药、糖皮质激素、细胞毒药物，缺点是副作用过大，包括胃肠道反应、肝肾毒性、感染、骨质疏松、骨髓抑制、胎儿致畸等。近年来，虽然生物制剂作为具有特异性的针对致病靶分子的拮抗药而成为治疗风湿类疾病的重要方向之一，但其价格昂贵，难以大规模推广。因此，大量风湿免疫系统疾病患者为缓解肢体关节疼痛症状会主动寻求中医药治疗。即使在西医院，雷公藤制剂等中成药也极为常用。

在中医学中，风湿性疾病属于"痹证"范畴。在病因上，中医学认为本病发于正气亏虚在先，而后受风、寒、湿等邪气侵入骨节经络而发病。在病机上，存在正气亏虚，风寒湿邪，或郁而化热，阻滞经络。在临床治疗上，以扶正祛邪为主要治疗大法。越来越多的临床证据表明，中医药在治疗风湿性疾病中，能够改善临床症状，减轻发作频次，减少不良反应，具有不可忽略的临床价值。本节将重点介绍类风湿性关节炎、系统性红斑狼疮、强直性脊柱炎、干燥综合征、雷诺病的中医认识及治疗。

二、风湿性疾病各论

1. 类风湿性关节炎

类风湿性关节炎是一种全身性自身免疫性疾病，以手和手腕等小关节的对称性、持续性及多发性的关节炎症为特征。临床表现有晨起关节僵硬，疼痛，肿胀，若不积极治疗，可造成关节畸形和功能丧失。常可累及心、肺、肾、神经系统等器官及组织，出现类风湿结节及血管炎、肺间质病变、心包炎、心肌炎和由于类风湿结节压迫而导致的多种神经系统表现。在我国，类风湿性发病率为 0.2% ~ 0.4%，任何年龄均可见，好发于 30 ~ 50 岁，女性与男性之比约为 3:1。

在病因上，感染及自身免疫反应是本病发生的中心环节，遗传、内分泌及环境因素可增加其易感性。发病机制主要为免疫紊乱。

在临床治疗上，常用药物包括非甾体抗炎药，抗风湿药，免疫抑制剂，糖皮质激素，生物制剂。甲氨蝶呤等为目前广泛使用的药物。然而，很多患者不耐受其伴随的胃肠道反应、肝肾毒性、感染、骨质疏松、骨髓抑制等不适。

在中医学中，本病属于"历节""尪痹"范畴。在病因病机上，为正气先虚，风、寒、湿、热等邪气阻滞经络。

在临床治疗中，常用中成药雷公藤多苷，以及经典名方麻黄加术汤、独活寄生汤。雷公藤多苷有"中草药激素"之称，是我国率先从卫矛科植物雷公藤根中提取研制的具有抗炎免疫调节作用的中药制剂。这是一种脂溶性混合物，其生理活性由二萜内酯、生物碱、三萜等多种有效成分协同叠加产生，既具有免疫抑制作用，又去除了毒性成分。在现今临床中，已被广泛运用于类风湿性关节炎、原发性肾小球肾病、肾病综合征、狼疮性肾炎、红斑狼疮、亚急性及慢性重症肝炎、慢性活动性肝炎等疾病的治疗。2012年，北京协和医院开展了雷公藤多苷治疗活动性类风湿性关节炎的随机对照临床研究，共纳入207例患者，研究发现，经过24周治疗，单用雷公藤多苷组取得55.1%的治疗有效率，高于单用甲氨蝶呤组的46.4%，而甲氨蝶呤与雷公藤多苷联合用药取得高达76.8%的治疗有效率。研究证实，对于活动性类风湿性关节炎，单用雷公藤多苷疗效不亚于单用甲氨蝶呤，两者联合使用疗效显著优于单用甲氨蝶呤，且不同药物组间的不良反应发生率无显著性差异。值得注意的是，长期服用雷公藤对性腺有一定毒性，未婚未育者慎用。用法用量：口服，每次按体重0.3~0.5mg/kg，一般为1~2片，一日3次餐后服用。

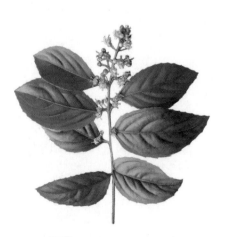

经典名方麻黄加术汤出自《金匮要略》，由麻黄、桂枝、杏仁、白术、甘草组成，具有散寒除湿，健脾温阳的功效。本方可用于类风湿性关节炎属风寒湿痹证的治疗。当患者临床表现为骨节疼痛，肿

雷公藤原植物图

胀，或有发热，食欲不振，苔白腻，脉浮紧，表证较明显，类似于感冒，遇寒加重时，就可以考虑运用本方。

独活寄生汤出自《备急千金要方》，由独活、桑寄生、秦艽、防风、细辛、川芎、当归、生地黄、白芍、肉桂、茯苓、杜仲、牛膝、人参、甘草组成。本方有祛风湿，止痹痛，益肝肾，补气血的功效。在治疗类风湿性关节炎时，如果伴肢体关节酸痛，遇冷加重，腰膝疼痛，酸软无力，肢节屈伸不利，畏寒喜温，心悸气短就可以考虑运用本方。

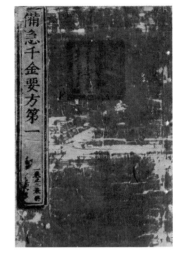

《备急千金要方》
中国中医科学院馆藏

参考文献

LYU Q W, ZHANG W, SHI Q, et al. Comparison of *Tripterygium wilfordii* Hook F. with methotrexate in the treatment of active rheumatoid arthritis (TRIFRA): a randomised, controlled clinical trial[J]. Annals of the Rheumatic Diseases, 2015, 74(6): 1-9.

2. 系统性红斑狼疮

系统性红斑狼疮是一种自身免疫病，是以免疫性炎症为突出表现的弥漫性结缔组织病，可导致人体多个器官、组织的损伤。在我国，其患病率为（30.13～70.41）/10万，其中育龄期女性多见，妊娠也能诱发。

其发病机制目前尚不明确，可能与遗传、内分泌及环境因素有关。环境因素可见于化学药品、病毒感染等。

在临床症状上，主要表现有面部特征性蝶形红斑，常见口或鼻黏膜溃疡，长期低、中度发热，对称性多关节疼痛、肿胀，但一般不会引起骨质损坏、偏头痛，严重者可见脑血管意外、癫痫、昏迷等。另外，还包括狼疮性肾炎、狼疮性肺炎、心包炎、肠炎、急性胰腺炎、结膜炎等全身各组织器官炎症。本病可因急性期多器官衰竭、感染而致死亡。

在临床治疗上，包括非甾体抗炎药、抗疟药、激素、免疫抑制剂、新型药物生物制剂、免疫球蛋白、血浆置换、造血干细胞移植等。然而，临床发现，部分患者不耐受上述治疗所带来的不良反应，包括消化道溃疡、出血、肝肾损伤、眼底病变、皮疹等。

在门诊，患者多为改善临床症状，减少并发症，减少副作用而寻求中医药治疗。

在中医学中，系统性红斑狼疮属于"阴阳毒""温毒发斑""蝶疮流浊"等范畴。在病因上，与感受外毒，先天不足，外内合邪，毒邪长期留滞体内损伤脏腑有关。在病机上，真阴不足为本，瘀毒痰阻为标。

在临床上，常用经典方犀角地黄汤及中成药白芍总苷胶囊。犀角地黄汤出自《外台秘要》，由犀角（现用水牛角代替）、地黄、芍药、牡丹皮组成，具有清热解毒，凉血散瘀的功效。现代药理学研究表明，本方具有镇静、抗惊厥、镇痛作用，可预防由系统性红斑狼疮引起的癫痫、昏迷等症状；本方对心血管系统、神经系统等多系统脏器具有保护作用，还具有抗炎、止血和提高免疫力等重要辅助作用，可改善狼疮引起的全身性器官损伤。芍药中白芍总苷具有抗炎和双向免疫调节作用，也是治疗此病的主要成分。红斑狼疮患者出现蝶形红斑、关节疼痛、身热、谵语、烦躁等症状时，可以考虑运用本方。

白芍总苷胶囊是从中药白芍中提取的多种具有生理功效成分的苷类混合物，由于其对免疫系统具有双向调节作用，现广泛用于类风湿性关节炎、系统性红斑狼疮、强直性脊柱炎等自身免疫疾病的辅助用药。一项共纳入 978 名红斑狼疮患者的针对白芍总苷在狼疮活动期的临床治疗研究表明，在 1~6 个月内该药可显著改善红斑狼疮活动度评分，之后会平稳维持和改善症状，并且能减少 24 小时尿蛋白，具有一定的肾脏保护作用。该药为天然药物提取物，尚未观察到相关不良反应，可长期服用。极少部分患者可能会有出现消化道症状，但多能自行缓解。用法用量：口服，一次 2 粒，一日 2~3 次。

参考文献

CHEN Y F, WANG L D, CAO Y, et al. Paeonia lactiflora total glucosides of for safely reducing disease activity in systemic lupus erythematosus: a systematic review and meta-analysis[J]. Front Pharmacol, 2022, 13: e834947. doi: 10. 3389/fphar. 2022. 834947.

3. 强直性脊柱炎

强直性脊柱炎是脊柱关节炎中以中轴脊柱关节受累为主的慢性炎症性风湿病，可伴有关节外表现，严重者可有脊柱强直和畸形。在病因上，该病是由遗传和环境因素共同作用所导致的多基因遗传病。本病具有很强的家族聚集性。环境因素主要与衣原体、沙门菌等肠道病原体感染激发机体炎症和免疫应答有关。在我国，其患病率在 0.25% 左右。男女比例 1∶1，男性病情较重。

在病理上，本病多表现为各个骨关节部位肌腱、韧带、关节囊等的反复性炎症、纤维化甚至骨化，多见于足跟、足掌、膝关节、胸肋、脊椎、髂嵴、股骨大转子、坐骨结节等处。

在临床症状上，早期表现为下腰背痛伴晨僵，或臀部、腹股沟向下肢放射性酸痛，活动后减轻。随病情进展可有腰椎及胸廓各方向活动受限。关节外症状可见虹膜炎、主动脉瓣病变，少数患者有肾功能异常、肺炎和肌肉萎缩。

在临床治疗上，本病一般不影响寿命，但致残率较高。该病对非甾体抗炎药反应良好，为临床一线用药。然而，本病病程较长，长期服用此类药物所带来的副作用常使患者难以忍受，故部分患者求助中医药治疗。

在中医学中，强直性脊柱炎属于"大偻""痹证"范畴。在病因上，与先天不足，外感湿毒有关。在病机上，以肾虚兼有湿热瘀阻为主。

在治疗上，常用经典名方金匮肾气丸、桂枝芍药知母汤标本兼治。

金匮肾气丸出自《金匮要略》，由地黄、山茱萸、山药、牡丹皮、泽泻、茯苓、桂枝、制附子组成，具有补肾助阳，化气行水的功效。临床可用于强直性脊柱炎患者伴腰膝酸软，畏寒肢冷，骨节疼痛，下肢水肿，小便不利等症状。药理学研究发现，金匮肾气丸具有调节免疫应答作用。该方常用于强直性脊柱炎缓解期。现已将本方研制成中成药水蜜丸剂型。用法用量：口服，每次 20（4g）~25 粒（5g），每日 2 次。

桂枝芍药知母汤出自《金匮要略》，由桂枝、芍药、知母、甘草、麻黄、生姜、白术、炮附子、防风组成，具有祛风除湿，散寒通阳的功效。现代药理学研究表明，桂枝芍药知母汤能够通过镇痛、抗炎、调节免疫等多方面改善症状，并且有保护骨关节，缓解骨关节损伤的作用。临床可用于治疗强直性脊柱炎缓解期患者伴见肢节疼痛，关节肿大，身体瘦弱，恶心呕吐，头晕目眩，脊柱及胸廓活动受限，舌淡红，苔薄白，脉弦细等。对强直性脊柱炎急性发作期也有良好的防治作用，临床可见关节"红、肿、热、痛"、活动功能障碍及由炎症引发的肾功能异常，血尿酸升高等表现。研究发现桂枝芍药知母汤能够保护肾功能，加快尿酸排出，抗炎镇痛。

4. 干燥综合征

干燥综合征是一种侵犯泪腺、唾液腺等外分泌腺体的慢性炎症性自身免疫系统疾病。在我国，干燥综合征患病率为 0.29％～0.77％，任何年龄可发，多见于 30～60 岁。

在病因及发病机制上，目前尚不明确，但遗传、感染、环境因素均参与其发病。主要病理反应为自身免疫反应和炎症介导的组织损伤，尤其是外分泌腺体。一般局限于外分泌腺体的预后较好，内脏损伤如治疗不及时可危及生命。

在临床表现上，包括干燥性角膜炎和口腔干燥症，可累及内脏器官，还会出现全身性表现，包括皮疹、关节痛、肾钙化、肾结石等肾病、干燥性咽喉炎、萎缩性胃炎、运动神经异常、偏瘫、血细胞减少、甲状腺炎、肺炎等多系统受累症状。

在临床治疗上，目前尚无根治方法。可用人工泪液、人工唾液及凝胶等腺体分泌物的替代治疗缓解症状，控制全身性自身免疫反应症状的免疫抑制剂，严重时加糖皮质激素，治疗肌肉、关节疼痛常用非甾体抗炎药，以及其他对症治疗。然而，我们发现，因需要终身用药，很多患者不耐受其副作用，为改善临床症状，提高生活质量，减轻副作用，常主动寻求中医药治疗。

在中医学中，干燥综合征属于"燥证""燥痹""燥毒"等范畴。在病因上，与先天禀赋不足，情志化火，外感燥邪，肝肾阴虚等有关。在病机上，以肝肾阴不足，气津亏虚，血瘀痹阻等有关。

在治疗上，经典方药一贯煎和杞菊地黄丸在临床极为常用。另外，若全身症状明显，多合用雷公藤多苷片或白芍总苷胶囊，对缓解症状、阻止病情发展具有重要意义。

一贯煎出自清代名医魏之琇的《续名医类案》，该方由地黄、北沙参、麦冬、当归、枸杞子、川楝子组成，具有滋阴疏肝的功效。临床多用于干燥综合征属肝肾阴虚，肝气郁滞证，表现为口燥咽干，舌红少津，胸胁疼痛。现代药理学研究表明一贯煎可以缓解腺体损伤，修复腺体的分泌功能。

杞菊地黄丸是在六味地黄丸的基础上加枸杞子和菊花而成，包括枸杞子、菊花、熟地黄、酒萸肉、牡丹皮、山药、茯苓、泽泻。该方可以滋肾养肝，用于干燥综合征肝肾阴亏，临床表现为畏光，目赤干涩，视物昏花，眩晕耳鸣等。现代药理学研究显示杞菊地黄丸具有较好的肾脏保护作用，对于预防干燥综合征诱导的各种严重肾损害有一定作用。杞菊地黄丸一般为浓缩丸，每 8 丸相当于原药材 3g，每瓶有 200 丸，每次口服 8 丸，每日 3 次。

5. 雷诺病

雷诺病是血管神经功能紊乱引起的肢端小动脉痉挛性疾病，不伴有全身系统性疾病表现，主要为原发性。继发性常作为症状出现在各种免疫疾病或结缔组织病、神经系统疾病、慢性闭塞性动脉疾病中，称为雷诺现象。本病多见于女性，男女比例 1∶10，好发年龄为 20～30 岁。雷诺病的主要表现为在寒冷或精神刺激等因素影响下，肢体远端皮肤如手掌出现对称性、阵发性的苍白、紫绀样改变、麻木及刺痛，保暖后转为潮红。

在病因上，雷诺病的发病原因尚不明确，目前认为主要与遗传、免疫、环境因素有关，寒冷及情绪刺激为其重要诱导因素，其他诱因有感染、疲劳等。初期雷诺病并不会引起严重后果。

在临床治疗上，可局部外用 2% 硝酸甘油软膏、复方肝素凝胶。系统用药有血管平滑肌松弛剂、周围血管扩张剂、5- 羟色胺拮抗剂等，若出现坏疽可能需手术截肢。自身免疫反应导致者常常病程漫长，预后差。并且由于自主神经功能紊乱，很多患者有失眠多梦、急躁易怒、郁闷等表现。此类患者多在西药控制基础上联合中医治疗，改善神经功能紊乱导致的各种症状，减轻副作用。

在中医学中，雷诺病属于"脉痹""血痹""厥证"等范畴。在病因上，与先天禀赋不足，阳虚受寒，情志不调等因素有关。在病机上，与脾肾阳虚，气血不足，寒邪痹阻，血行不畅有关。

在临床治疗中，常用经典名方阳和汤和黄芪桂枝五物汤。阳和汤出自《外科证治全生集》，由熟地黄、鹿角胶、姜炭、肉桂、麻黄、白芥子、生甘草组成。本方具有温阳补血，散寒通滞的功效。可用于雷诺病伴紫绀或苍白，遇寒加重，麻木疼痛，口中不渴，舌淡苔白，脉沉细。尤其有坏疽倾向时可使用。现代药理学研究显示，阳和汤具有降低炎症因子水平和氧化应激水平，减轻神经性炎症的作用，对周围神经病变性疾病及免疫系统疾病疗效良好。

黄芪桂枝五物汤出自《金匮要略》，由黄芪、桂枝、芍药、生姜、大枣组成，具有温经通络、活血止痛、益气固卫功效。现代药理学研究也表明，该方具有抗炎、镇痛、保护血管内皮、增强免疫等作用，对周围神经病变具有良好的疗效。雷诺病伴见有疲倦乏力、汗多、心慌烦躁、头晕耳鸣、肢端麻木或有疼痛，舌暗红，脉虚或弦等症状可选用本方。

第八节
神经系统疾病

一、神经系统疾病概述

很多人曾经都有过突然手麻、腿麻、肢体抖动的经历，这些临床症状可能都与神经系统疾病有关。所谓的神经系统疾病，是包括发生在中枢神经系统、周围神经系统以及自主神经系统的病症，同时也以可表现为意识障碍、感觉障碍、运动障碍、肌张力异常等，其中运动障碍可有瘫痪、非自主运动等表现。

神经系统疾病的病变范围非常广泛，涉及全身的神经部位。临床常见的神经系统疾病包括脑梗死、短暂性脑缺血发作、脑出血、肌萎缩侧索硬化、帕金森病、癫痫、进行性肌营养不良、共济失调等。值得注意的是，神经系统疾病非常复杂，在临床上或难以诊断，或难以治疗，且因神经系统疾病导致的高致死率和致残率，患者的功能恢复问题已经成为现今临床公认的医学难题。

中医学对于神经系统疾病的病因病机有着独特的认知体系。中医学认为，其与风邪密切相关，包括内风与外风两种类型。这在《黄帝内经》中就有专门论述，包括"邪风""击仆""偏枯"。在《金匮要略·中风历节病脉证并治》中也指出："夫风之为病，当半身不遂，或但臂不遂者，此为痹。脉微而数，中风使然。"在治疗上，中医药在促进患者肢体功能恢复、改善生活质量上，也具有一定的疗效。本节讨论中医药对脑梗死、头晕的认识与临床诊疗方案。

二、神经系统疾病各论

1. 脑梗死

脑梗死，又称缺血性脑卒中，是指因各种原因导致脑动脉血流中断，局部脑组织缺氧、缺血性坏死，从而导致相应神经功能缺损的脑血管病。脑梗死大约占全部脑卒中的80%。脑梗死常见的原因包括动脉粥样硬化、心源性栓塞、小动脉闭塞等。在临床上，常见的脑梗死类型包括脑血栓、腔隙性脑梗死和脑栓塞。该病不仅给人类健康带来较大威胁，也给患者及社会带来了沉重的负担。

在临床症状上，本病多见于45~70岁中老年人，常急性起病，症状的严重程度与脑损害的部位、脑缺血性血管大小、缺血的严重程度有关，轻者可无任何症状，重者可表现为神经功能障碍，包括猝然昏倒、不省人事、半身不遂、言语障碍、智力障碍、偏盲、头晕、面瘫、共济失调、大小便失禁等。

在临床诊断上，需结合患者既往病史、临床表现，以及脑 CT、MRI、经颅多普勒超声、颈动脉彩色 B 超、磁共振、血管造影、数字减影全脑血管造影、颈动脉造影等，即可明确诊断。

在临床治疗上，包括急性期溶栓、血管内介入、抗栓、抗凝、扩容，以及规范化二级预防药物治疗。脑梗死的预后不同，一般小血管闭塞的预后比较好。

值得注意的是，本病是一种高致残率及高致死率的疾病，其溶栓治疗具有严格的时间窗，很多患者在就医时已经错过溶栓的最佳时机，部分患者对阿司匹林、他汀等药物不耐受，或由于西药的不良反应等问题，在一定程度上限制了其临床运用。而在脑梗死急性期以及恢复期，通过包括针灸在内的中医药早期干预，在一定程度上，能够改善肢体功能，促进恢复，提高生活质量，减少病死率。

脑梗死属于中医学的"中风"范畴。在病因上，多由于正气虚亏、饮食不节、情志失调、劳倦内伤等引起气血逆乱，进而导致风、火、痰、瘀等病理因素内生，痹阻经络。根据神志受损程度的不同，本病有中经络、中脏腑之分。

在临床中，急性期可早期运用经典名方安宫牛黄丸，在恢复期可配合针灸、推拿等治疗措施。安宫牛黄丸出自清代医家吴鞠通的《温病条辨》，为中医著名的"凉开三宝"之一，为脑梗死急性期的急救良药。该药由牛黄、水牛角浓缩粉、人工麝香、珍珠、朱砂、雄黄、黄连、黄芩、栀子、郁金、冰片组成，可以清热解毒，镇惊开窍。在脑梗死急性期，如果见到高热烦躁，惊厥，神昏谵语，牙关紧闭，半身不遂，面红目赤，呼吸气粗，喉间痰鸣，舌红，脉滑，这就属于典型的"邪入心包"，就可以考虑运用本方。

针灸、推拿等传统中医理疗手段对脑梗死导致的肢体不遂、言语不利、失眠、麻木疼痛、肌肉痉挛或痿软等后遗症具有独特疗效。在辨证选穴上，头部穴位常选百会、四神聪、神庭、印堂、太阳、风池；合并言语不利，或者吞咽障碍，常选承浆、廉泉；合并中枢性面瘫，常选地仓、颊车；在四肢穴位上，上肢可取曲池、手三里、外关、内关、神门、合谷、后溪；下肢可取血海、梁丘、阴陵泉、阳陵泉、足三里、上巨虚、下巨虚、三阴交、解溪、照海、昆仑、太冲、太白。

参考文献

熊兴江. 古代"中风"内涵及《千金要方》小续命汤治疗脑梗死、脑出血体会 [J]. 中国中药杂志，2020，45（12）：2735-2751.

2. 头晕

我们在门诊时见到，很多人都会因为突然发现头晕不能自主，甚至不能站立，怀疑自己是不是得了脑梗死？是不是出了什么大问题？这在老年人中尤其常见。前来门诊就诊检查后，很多时候都会考虑这是由于混合性原因导致的，可能与脑梗死、脑动脉供血不足、颈椎病等多种疾病有关。在临床上，头晕到底是怎么一回事？是由哪些疾病导致的？

头晕是临床常见的症状，可表现为头昏、头胀、头重脚轻、眼花，也可伴有乏力、失眠、耳鸣、健忘等不适。导致头晕的原因比较复杂，包括脑缺血、脑外伤、脑动脉硬化、椎－基底动脉供血不足、神经衰弱、高血压、低血压、颈椎病、低血糖、癫痫、贫血、感染、中毒、梅尼埃病、心律失常、心力衰竭、自主神经功能紊乱、药物中毒等。

在临床诊断时，针对头晕患者，在详细了解病史和全面体格检查基础上，可行前庭功能、眼底、心电图、脑电图，以及头颅、颈椎 CT 检查等以排查病因。

在中医学中，头晕属于"头风""眩晕"等范畴。在病因上，与情志内伤、饮食不节、头部外伤或手术、体虚、久病、失血、劳倦过度等密切相关。在病机上，与气血亏虚、肾精不足导致脑髓空虚，清窍失养，或肝阳上亢、痰火上逆、瘀血阻窍导致清窍上扰有关。

在临床治疗中，常用经典名方泽泻汤与归脾汤。泽泻汤出自张仲景的《金匮要略》。该方由泽泻、白术组成，具有利水除饮、健脾制水功效。在古代，这张处方主治"心下有支饮，其人苦冒眩"。就是说，患者表现为头目眩晕，属于水饮导致，就可以考虑用这张处方。我们现在用它来治疗脑梗死、高血压、颈椎病、脑供血不足等各种疾病引起的头晕，可以显著改善头晕症状。我们曾经治疗过一例颈椎病合并脑供血不足的头晕患者，不能下地行走，服用泽泻汤后当天头就不晕，类似的经验还有很多。

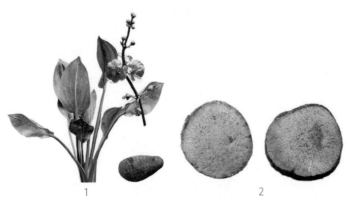

泽泻原植物及饮片图

1. 原植物；2. 泽泻饮片。

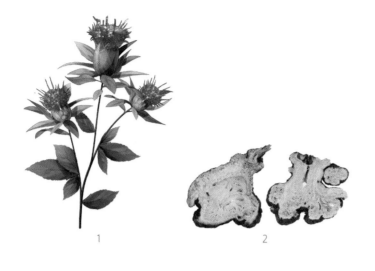

白术原植物及饮片图
1. 原植物；2. 白术饮片。

归脾汤也是一张经典名方，出自《正体类要》。归脾汤由白术、人参、黄芪、当归、甘草、茯苓、远志、酸枣仁、木香、龙眼肉、生姜、大枣等中药组成，具有益气补血、健脾养心功效。对于头晕患者表现为容易心慌心悸，失眠，健忘，盗汗，倦怠乏力，纳差，面色萎黄没有光泽，舌淡，苔薄白，脉细弱，就可以考虑选择运用本方。我们发现，一般低血压及体质虚弱患者，常能有用到本方的机会。中成药归脾丸就是出自于归脾汤，常用的服用方法为口服，用温开水或生姜汤送服，水蜜丸每次 6g，小蜜丸每次 9g，大蜜丸每次 1 丸，每日 3 次。

当然，头晕的类型很多，还有高血压导致的头晕，在治疗上会选择相应既能改善头晕，又能降压的中药；针对自主神经功能紊乱、焦虑、抑郁的患者，还需要针对其焦虑状态，选择相应的中药。

第九节
恶性肿瘤

一、恶性肿瘤概述

恶性肿瘤，又称癌症。一提到癌症，许多人都会谈之色变，甚至不少医生也认为它是不可攻克的医学难题。据 2019 年世界卫生组织统计，癌症是全球大部分国家人口的第一或第二大死因，为各国带来了沉重的疾病负担。据 2022 年我国国家癌症中心最新统计报告，2016 年我国新发癌症病例 406.4 万例，世标发病率 186.46/10 万，男性发病率明显高于女性。2016 年我国癌症总死亡人数 241.4 万，世标死亡率 105.19/10 万，男性死亡率几乎比女性高出 1 倍。肺癌、肝癌、胃癌是导致死亡人数最多的三种癌症，占所有癌症死亡人数的四成以上。

癌症在早期可不伴有明显症状，如早期肺癌、肝癌、胃癌，常通过 CT、内镜等检查时偶然发现。随着病情进展，肿瘤增大或侵袭其他组织器官时，就可能出现明显消瘦、痰中带血、进行性吞咽困难、黄疸、疼痛等症状。在临床治疗上，常选择化疗、放疗、手术切除、靶向治疗、生物治疗等方式综合干预。积极治疗可以使 30% 以上的癌症得到根治，对于延缓癌症进展、延长患者生命具有重要作用。然而，我们也发现，部分患者或因不耐受放化疗副作用，或因畏惧手术，或因癌症晚期多发转移，而希望寻求中医或中西医结合治疗以"增效减毒"，达到更好的治疗效果。

癌症在中医学中属于"癌病""积聚类病"等范畴。在病因病机上多因正气虚弱、外感邪毒、情志内伤、饮食不节等导致脏腑功能失调、气血津液运行不畅而致痰、瘀、毒等内生，相互搏结，久而成癌。近年来，中药在减轻放化疗不良反应、缓解癌症相关症状、抑制肿瘤增大和转移、提高患者免疫力与机体功能、改善患者生命质量等方面发挥了积极的作用，中医药治疗癌症的临床价值越来越受到国内外认可。本节将重点讨论中医药治疗肺癌、肝癌、胃癌三种癌症的中医认识与临床诊疗方案。

二、恶性肿瘤各论

1. 肺癌

在临床上我们常见到一些吸烟的中老年男性，出现迁延不愈的咳嗽、咳带血痰液，然而他们未予重视，直至出现显著胸痛、咯血、消瘦，才去医院检查，却发现已是晚期肺癌。据统计，2020 年全球有超过 200 万人患上肺癌，有近

180 万人因肺癌而死去。肺癌也是我国每年新发与死亡病例数最多的恶性肿瘤，给社会和患者家庭带来沉重负担。

吸烟是导致肺癌的最常见因素，吸烟使肺癌发生的风险平均高出 10 倍。除吸烟外，空气污染、不良的工作环境、不健康的生活方式也是导致肺癌的重要原因。

在临床表现上，早期肺癌可不出现任何症状，但随着病情进展，肿瘤侵袭支气管、血管等，可出现咳嗽、痰中带血甚至咯血等。中晚期肺癌患者可出现明显消瘦、咳嗽、咯血、气短、胸痛、乏力、发热、声嘶等症状。

在临床诊断上，胸部 X 线、CT、MRI 等影像学检查是发现肺癌最重要的手段，许多早期肺癌都是由此被发现。另外，痰脱落细胞学检查、呼吸内镜检查、肺组织病理学检查都是诊断肺癌的重要手段。

在临床治疗上，主要包括手术治疗、药物治疗及放射治疗等。中医药在协同增效，减轻放化疗不良反应，提高免疫力和机体功能，改善生活质量等方面，具有很高的临床价值。因此，许多患者往往主动寻求中医药治疗。

肺癌属于中医学"肺积""息贲"等范畴。在病因上与禀赋不足、正气虚损、邪毒侵肺、痰湿内聚等有关，其主要病机为正虚不能御邪，痰湿、邪毒等侵袭肺脏，肺失宣降、气血壅滞、痰毒瘀相互搏结，久则发为肺癌。

在临床治疗上，可选择经典名方麦门冬汤和中药注射剂艾迪注射液。麦门冬汤是汉代医圣张仲景创制的千古名方，由麦冬、半夏、人参、甘草、粳米、大枣 6 味中药组成，具有益气养阴、化痰散结的功效。由于部分肺癌症状与原书中描述的"肺痿"表现相似，所以麦门冬汤也被用来治疗以咳嗽、气急、咽喉不适、咳浊唾涎沫、胸痛、痰中带血、舌红、苔少、脉虚数等气阴两虚表现为主的肺癌患者。在运用时，可酌加鳖甲、半枝莲、白花蛇舌草等具有抗癌散结作用的中药以增强疗效。

艾迪注射液是一种具有抗癌作用的中药注射剂，它由人参、黄芪、刺五加、斑蝥 4 味中药组成，具有清热解毒、消瘀散结的功效。艾迪注射液可用于原发性肝癌、肺癌、鼻咽癌等各类肿瘤术后的巩固治疗。临床上也常将它与化疗药物配合使用，能够起到增效减毒的作用。一项纳入 4053 名非小细胞肺癌患者、共 54 项临床试验的系统评价发现，艾迪注射液联合西药化疗方案，能显著提高临床缓解率和疾病控制率，减轻骨髓抑制、中性粒细胞减少、血小板减少、贫血、胃肠道反应，改善肝功能。现代药理学研究发现，艾迪注射液能较好地抑制实体瘤，增强人体免疫力和机体功能，此外还能减轻化疗导致的骨髓抑制，维持白细胞和血小板的正常水平。

参考文献

XIAO Z, JIANG Y, WANG C Q, et al. Clinical efficacy and safety of aidi injection combination with vinorelbine and cisplatin for advanced non-small-cell lung carcinoma: a systematic review and meta-analysis of 54 randomized controlled trials[J]. Pharmacol Res, 2020, 153: 104637. doi: 10.1016/j. phrs. 2020. 104637.

2. 肝癌

酗酒？吸烟？总是吃霉变食物？肝炎不积极治疗？如果有这些行为，肝癌可能很快找上门。2020 年我国肝癌新发病例数超过 450 万，占全球的 20% 以上，死亡人数超过 300 万，占全球的 30% 以上。此外，男性发病率约为女性的 3 倍。

在病因上，乙肝病毒感染导致的病毒性肝炎是我国肝癌发病的主要原因，经常食用黄曲霉毒素污染的食物、酗酒等导致肝纤维化及肝硬化、长期接触有毒化学物质等是肝癌发生的重要原因。

在临床表现上，肝癌起病隐匿，早期无明显症状，当症状明显时往往已是中、晚期阶段。中晚期肝癌常出现持续性肝区胀痛或钝痛、肝脏进行性增大且质地变硬以及黄疸、消瘦、纳差等全身症状。

在临床诊断上，肝脏组织病理检查可明确诊断，肝癌标志物如甲胎蛋白是诊断肝癌的特异标志物，B 超、增强 CT 和 MRI 也在肝癌的早期诊断及病情评估等方面发挥重要作用。

在临床治疗上，包括手术、肝脏移植、射频消融、微波消融以及靶向治疗等。不少患者为求得更好疗效，往往也会寻求中医药的帮助。

肝癌属于中医学"癥瘕""肥气""臌胀"等范畴。在病因上，与正气亏虚、脏腑虚损、七情郁结、邪毒侵袭等相关。在病机上，脏腑阴阳失调，气血津液运行不畅，肝失疏泄，导致痰毒瘀相互搏结，久则发为肝癌。

在临床治疗上，可选用经典名方鳖甲煎丸和中药注射剂康莱特注射液。鳖甲煎丸出自汉代医圣张仲景所著的《金匮要略》，由鳖甲、射干、黄芩、柴胡、鼠妇、干姜、大黄、芍药、桂枝、葶苈子、石韦、厚朴、牡丹皮、瞿麦、凌霄花、半夏、人参、蜈蚣、土鳖虫、蜂房、阿胶、硝石、桃仁 23 味中药组成，具有活血化瘀、软坚散结的功效，适用于肝癌中晚期出现肝脏质地坚硬、表面凹凸、多发结节等情况。在运用时，可以适当增加一些具有抗癌散结作用的中药，如半枝莲、白花蛇舌草等。鳖甲煎丸已被研制成中成药，它为黑褐色水蜜丸，每次口服 3g，一日 3 次。

康莱特注射液是由中药薏苡仁提取而成。薏苡仁为禾本科植物薏米的干燥成熟种仁，味甘、淡，性微寒，归脾、胃、肺经，具有利湿、健脾、除痹、清热排脓的功效。康莱特注射液有益气养阴，消癥散结的功效，适用于原发性肝癌和非小细胞肺癌，经中医辨证属于气阴两虚证患者。现代药理学研究发现，它可以明显增强免疫力，抑制肿瘤细胞生长，使肿瘤细胞变性。康莱特注射液以缓慢静脉滴注的方式给药，每日 1 次，每次 200ml，三周为一个疗程。

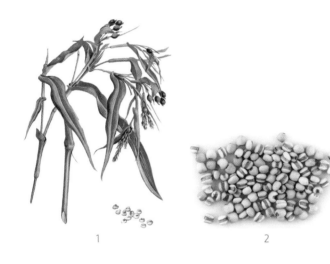

薏苡仁原植物及饮片图
1.原植物；2.薏苡仁饮片。

3. 胃癌

在临床上，经常见到患有慢性萎缩性胃炎、胃溃疡、胃息肉等疾病的患者，由于未能进行积极治疗最后进展成为胃癌，为家庭和个人带来极大痛苦。

2020 年中国胃癌新发病例数约 47.9 万，占全国癌症新发病例数的 10.5%，死亡病例数约 37.4 万，占癌症总死亡人数 12.4%。全球 43.9% 的胃癌新发病例和 48.6% 的胃癌致死病例发生在我国。

在病因上，幽门螺杆菌感染、慢性萎缩性胃炎、肠上皮化生及吸烟、遗传是胃癌发生的高风险因素。在多致病因素的综合作用下出现"炎 - 癌转化"，最终导致胃癌的发生。

在临床表现上，80% 的早期胃癌患者无任何症状，部分可出现消化不良。随着病情进展，许多患者可能出现消瘦、上腹部疼痛、贫血、纳差、黑便等症状。

在临床诊断上，胃镜检查结合组织活检是诊断胃癌、评估病情的最可靠方法。此外，肿瘤标志物和影像学检查也可辅助诊断。

在临床治疗上，根据病情，可采取包括内镜治疗、手术切除、化疗等手段。然而，部分患者因存在严重的不良反应，不耐受放化疗等治疗，主动寻求中医药治疗，以改善临床不适，延缓胃癌进展，提高生活质量，延长生存期。

在中医学中，胃癌属于"胃脘痛""噎膈"等范畴。在病因上，与脾胃虚弱、饮食不当、虫毒侵扰、情志内伤等关系密切。在病机上，脾胃虚弱，气机升降失调，加之痰浊、虫毒、瘀血等流于胃腑，相互搏结，则发为胃癌。

在临床治疗上，常选用经典名方半夏泻心汤和中药注射剂华蟾素注射液。半夏泻心汤出自医圣张仲景所著的《伤寒论》，由半夏、黄连、黄芩、人参、干姜、大枣、甘草 7 味中药组成，具有平调寒热、消痞散结功效，被誉为"胃肠病第一方"。半夏泻心汤在治疗胃癌癌前病变、调节胃癌微环境、抑制肿瘤生长以及缓解胃痛、胃胀、反酸、纳差、消化不良等方面具有一定作用。在临床运用时，可酌情配伍具有抗癌作用的中药，如半枝莲、白花蛇舌草、山慈菇、鬼箭羽等。

华蟾素注射液是以中华大蟾蜍的阴干全皮为原料，加工而成的一种具有抗癌作用的中药注射剂。蟾皮具有清热解毒、利水消肿的功效，可用于痈疽、瘰疬、肿瘤等疾病。一项纳入 1939 例胃癌晚期患者、共 27 项临床试验的荟萃分析表明，与单用化疗相比，联合华蟾素不但可显著提高总体缓解率与疾病控制率，而且能缓解化疗导致的恶心呕吐、腹泻、白细胞减少、周围神经毒性等不良反应。现代药理学研究发现，华蟾素可抑制肿瘤细胞增殖、诱导肿瘤细胞凋亡并可抑制肿瘤新生血管形成。

参考文献

SUN H, WANG W, BAI M, et al. Cinobufotalin as an effective adjuvant therapy for advanced gastric cancer: a meta-analysis of randomized controlled trials[J]. Onco Targets Ther, 2019, 12: 3139-3160.

第三章

中医临床诊疗展望

习近平强调"要遵循中医药发展规律，传承精华，守正创新"。中医学中有很多学术流派、学术观点，但不全是"精华"，但中医学的经典著作《伤寒论》以及后世中医名家流传下来的行之有效的方剂一定是中医学的"精华"所在。因此，我们常将医圣张仲景《伤寒论》中的经方，以及后世广为流传、广为运用的方剂统称为经典名方。比如我们所熟悉的治疗发热用的小柴胡汤/颗粒，治疗急性支气管炎和肺炎用的麻杏石甘汤/片，治疗女性胸胁胀痛、乳腺结节的逍遥丸/颗粒，治疗肾虚腰痛的六味地黄丸和肾气丸等。与现今临床常用的自拟方相比，经典名方无论在有效性还是安全性上都相对优越。现代临床运用的大量中成药、中药注射剂都来自于经典名方。

"创新"是指我们在传统中医药理论指导下，将中药、针灸、推拿等中医的治疗手段和方法运用于解决当前的临床医学难题。很多人可能会认为，西医学已经这么先进了，还会存在不能解决的临床难题吗？其实，在临床我们会遇到大量的西医学无能为力的病症。首先，新型冠状病毒感染就是一个鲜明的例子，中医药和中西医结合在治疗过程中发挥了重要作用（Pharmacol Res 2020）。除此之外，各种病毒感染性疾病，包括甲流、SARS 等，抗病毒及对症支持治疗疗效不佳。其次，在大量疾病的前期阶段，包括高血压前期、糖尿病前期（糖耐量异常）、癌前病变、肺部结节（< 8mm）等疾病，西医学尚缺乏有效治疗手段。再次，某些疾病如风湿免疫系统疾病等，西医学常规采用免疫抑制剂和激素，然而存在疗效有限，副作用较大，患者不耐受等问题。最后，在功能性疾病方面，包括自主神经功能紊乱、心脏神经官能症，甚至一些令患者饱受痛苦但检查却未见显著异常的病症，中医药具有确切的疗效。

可喜的是，近年来，中医药的临床优势逐渐受到国际认可。我国在天芪降糖胶囊治疗糖耐量减低、针刺治疗混合性尿失禁、女性压力性尿失禁、慢性难治性便秘、慢性前列腺炎/慢性盆底痛综合征、良性前列腺增生症，麻仁丸治疗便秘，中医药治疗溃疡性结肠炎，太极拳治疗类风湿性关节炎等方面逐渐取得高质量临床证据。另外，在头晕、失眠、焦虑等病症方面，虽然尚未取得高质量证据，但在临床已经取得较好疗效，同样值得关注。

TCM Clinical
Diagnosis and
Treatment

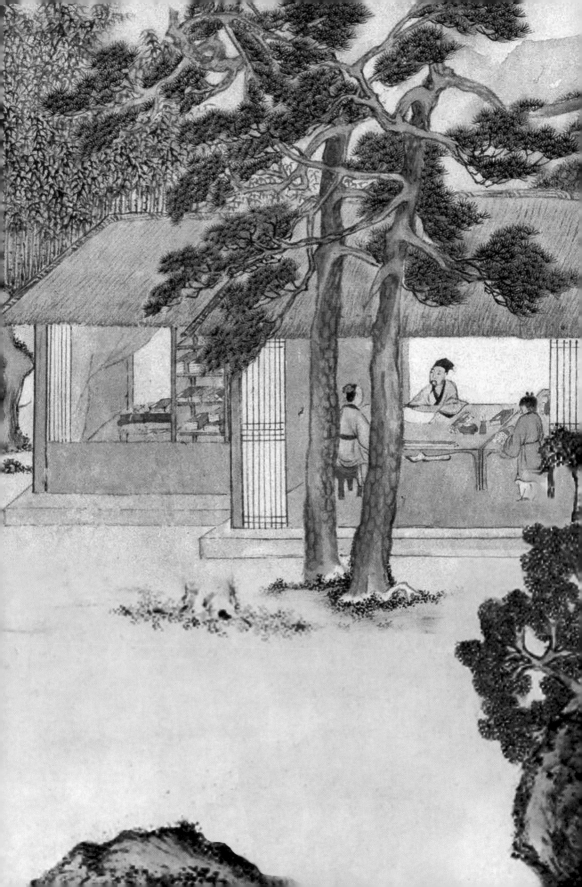

Chapter 1

The Introduction of

TCM and Therapy

Section 1
Medicine Therapy

I Chinese medicinals

Under the guidance of Chinese traditional medicine theory, Chinese medicinals are used to prevent, treat and diagnose diseases by collecting, processing and preparing medicinal materials, which have the functions of rehabilitation and health care and can guide the clinical application of traditional Chinese medicine and pharmacy. Chinese medicinals mainly come from natural medicine and their processed products, including plant medicines, animal medicines, mineral medicines and some chemical and biological products. "All medicines are based on herbs". Among these 5 subcategories, botanical medicines are especially common in Chinese medicine.

Here the clinical application of single medicinal, effective components and dietary supplements is emphatically introduced. The treatment of single Chinese medicinal has been recorded in ancient times, which belongs to the "medicinal used singly" of the seven emotions of compatibility of Chinese medicinals. *Shennong's Classic of Materia Medica–Preface* sums up the compatibility of various medicinals as "there is medicine used singly, or for mutual promotion, mutual enhancement, incompatibility, mutual inhibition, antagonism, and counteractive toxicity of another medicine. All these seven emotions are considered in harmony". It also records, "the solitary prescription is single prescription which does not need an adjuvant". Medicinal used singly is the clinical use of one Chinese medicinal to treat a single disease. In the face of simple diseases, choosing a medicinal with strong pertinence can achieve the therapeutic purpose. In *Treatise on Cold Pathogenic Diseases*, there are 4 prescriptions using single medicinal to treat diseases, including article 141 Wen'ge Powder (Wen'ge) in Taiyang disease, article 233 Mijiandao Formula (Honey) in Yangming disease, article 311 Gancao Decoction in Shaoyin disease, and article 392 Shaokun Powder in yin-yang deficiency caused by fatigue after illness. In ancient times, Dushen Decoction was used to treat critical patients with the collapse of yuan qi caused by massive blood loss with Renshen (Ginseng Radix et Rhizoma) alone; Qingjin Powder used Huangqin (Scutellariae Radix) to treat hemoptysis caused by lung heat. Others include: *Shennong's Classic of*

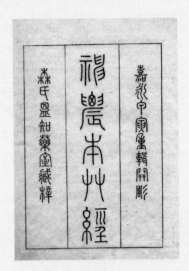

Shen Nong's Classic of the Materia Medica
(Shén Nóng Běn Cǎo Jīng, 神农本草经)

Materia Medica records that Chinese medicine, Huanglian (Coptidis Rhizoma), is used to treat diarrhea; Machixian (Portulacae Herba) treats dysentery; Xiakucao (Prunellae Spica) Ointments treat goiter tumor; Yimucao (Leonuri Herba) Ointments promote blood circulation for regulating menstruation and removing obstruction in collaterals and relieving pain; Xianhecao (Agrimoniae Herba) destroys and expels tenia, which are effective methods of clinical treatment.

Effective ingredients of Chinese medicinals refer to monomer compounds derived from Chinese medicinals, which play a role in biological metabolism or chemical reaction, and play a major pharmacodynamic role in Chinese medicinal materials. Effective ingredients can generally be expressed by molecular formula and structural formula, such as ephedrine and artemisinin. This research idea of screening new chemical medicines from natural medicines has made remarkable achievements in the research process in recent decades. For example, artemisinin is for treating malaria, paclitaxel for anti-tumor, levo ephedrine for relieving spasm and calming panting, salvianolate for promoting blood circulation, removing blood stasis, and removing obstruction in collaterals and relieving pain, tanshinone II_A sodium sulfonate for promoting blood circulation and removing obstruction in collaterals, etc.

Dietary supplements are derived from natural medicines or produced by chemical or biotechnology, including animal and plant extracts, vitamins, minerals, amino acids, dietary fiber and so on. In the United States, the concept of dietary supplement originated from the *Dietary Supplements Health and Education Act* (DSHEA) promulgated by the U.S. Food and Drug Administration in 1994. Dietary supplements generally take tablets or capsules as the main dosage forms. Through oral dietary supplements, the necessary nutrients and bioactive substances are supplemented to promote the health of the body and reduce the onset of diseases. Generally speaking, the active substances contained in dietary supplements have a clear structure, stable physical and chemical properties and clear action mechanism. Dietary supplements are especially common in clinical applications nowadays. A large number of Chinese medicinals are classified as dietary supplements, including allicin, monascus, ginkgo leaf preparations and so on.

‖ Classic prescriptions

Classic prescriptions refer to TCM prescriptions that have been tempered clinically for thousands of years under the guidance of TCM theory. Because they originate from ancient classic medical books or representative ancient TCM works, they have a definite clinical curative effect, have been widely used by TCM doctors in the past dynasties, and have been used up to now. In today's clinical practice, classic prescriptions have been widely used in the treatment of diseases in various clinical departments, including Maxing Shigan Decoction for pneumonia, Tianma Gouteng Decoction for hypertension, Zhigancao Decoction for myocarditis, Banxia Xiexin Decoction for chronic gastritis, Xiaochaihu Decoction for infectious fever, Zhengan Xifeng Decoction for acute cerebral infarction and so on.

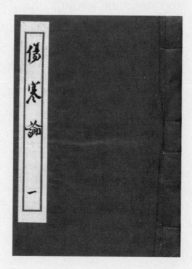

Treatise on Cold Pathogenic Diseases (Shāng Hán Lùn, 伤寒论)
Preserved in China Academy of Chinese Medical Sciences (CACMS)

III Chinese patent medicines

Chinese patent medicines refer to Chinese medicine products of different dosage forms processed according to certain principles, including pills, powders, ointments and min-pills. Chinese patent medicine has a long history of application, which is the essence of effective prescriptions summarized by TCM doctors through thousands of years of clinical practice. Chinese patent medicine can be divided into oral and external use. Commonly used dosage forms of oral Chinese patent medicine include pills, powders, granules, tablets, capsules, etc., which can be used for various diseases caused by dysfunction of qi, blood and zang-fu viscera. Commonly used dosage forms of Chinese patent medicine for external use include ointment paste, tincture, liniment, suppository, nasal drops, eye drops, aerosol, etc., which can be used for various diseases in surgery, orthopedics, dermatology and ENT. Chinese patent medicines can be widely used in clinical because of their fixed composition and wide application, but their deficiency is not free to add or subtract.

According to the clinical efficacy of medicines, Chinese patent medicines can be divided into exterior-relieving, purgation, heat-clearing, interior-warming, supplementing, tranquillizing, astringing, qi-regulating, blood-regulating, dampness-eliminating, wind-dispelling, phlegm-expelling, cough-relieving and panting-calming, digestion-promoting, etc. Chinese patent medicines are widely used in clinical practice, such as Suxiao Jiuxin Pill for angina pectoris of coronary heart disease, Naoliqing Pill for dizziness and headache of cerebral infarction, Huoxiang Zhengqi Soft Capsule for acute and chronic gastroenteritis and gastrointestinal cold, Xiaoyao Granule for distending pain in chest and hypochondrium and irregular menstruation of women, Guizhi Fuling Pill for gynecological uterine fibroids, Huoxue Zhitong Paste for joint pain, etc.

Section 2
Non–medicine Therapy

| Acupuncture

Acupuncture therapy means that under the guidance of TCM theory, needles (usually filiform needles) are pierced into patients at a certain angle, and acupuncture techniques, such as twirling, lifting and thrusting of the needle are comprehensively used to stimulate specific parts (acupoints) of the human body, which has the effects of activating collaterals and promoting blood circulation for removing blood stasis, so as to achieve the purpose of treating diseases. The piercing points are called human acupoints, referred to as acupoints for short.

According to different acupuncture shapes, uses and stimulation methods, acupuncture therapy can be divided into the following types: filiform needle therapy, cutaneous needle therapy, intradermal needle therapy, fire needle therapy, water needle therapy, Chi needle therapy, electroacupuncture therapy, pricking therapy, round-sharp needle therapy and so on. Acupuncture therapy has the advantages of wide indications, remarkable curative effect, simple and convenient operation, safety and economy, which is well received by clinicians and patients.

Taking cardiovascular diseases as an example, as the most widely used non-medicine therapy in TCM, acupuncture can not only improve the clinical discomfort symptoms, such as chest oppression, dizziness, headache and palpitation in patients with coronary heart disease, hypertension and arrhythmia, but also reduce the frequency of attacks, steadily reduce blood pressure, complications and target organ damage, which has certain clinical value and significance.

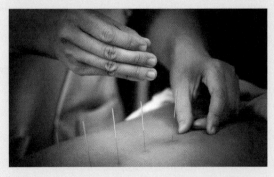

Acupuncture manipulation

|| Tai Chi

Tai Chi is a traditional martial art, which is also a sport and fitness project and has a long history in China. Tai Chi is a set of kungfu created according to the principle of yin and yang in the ancient *Book of Changes*, the meridian theory of TCM, Taoist daoyin, and exhalation and inhalation, which has the nature of yin and yang, conforms to human body structure and the operation law of nature. Tai Chi combines the traditional theory of yin and yang and the five elements of our country. Through the combination and transformation of movement and stillness, it promotes the circulation of qi and blood in the zang-fu viscera, improves the function of the zang-fu organs, and keeps the body and mind in a harmonious balance. In modern clinical practice, Tai Chi is also widely used in the treatment and rehabilitation of various chronic diseases, including chronic obstructive pulmonary disease, hypertension, coronary heart disease, cerebral infarction, Parkinson's disease and other diseases.

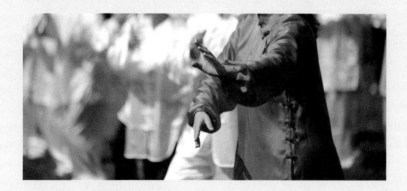

Tai Chi

||| Baduanjin

Baduanjin originated in the Northern Song Dynasty and has a history of more than 800 years. According to the description in *A Collection of Strange Things by Yi Jian* written by Hong Mai in the Northern Song Dynasty, "in the 7th year of Zhenghe, Li Siju held the office of recording the emperor's words and deeds ... who was good at exhalation and inhalation and massage, doing the so-called Baduanjin". Baduanjin has a total of 8 movements, including lifting hands up to dredge Sanjiao, opening the bow left and right like shooting a carving, raising one hand to regulate the spleen and stomach, looking back to treat five consumptions and seven damages, shaking head and swinging tail to remove the heart fire, bending down and touching feet with both hands to strengthen kidney and waist, making fists and opening eyes angrily to increase strength, and tiptoeing 7 times to eliminate all diseases. In ancient times, this set of movements was compared to "brocade", which means colorful, beautiful and luxurious.

Compared with strenuous exercise, Baduanjin requires less physical strength. It is widely used in the treatment and rehabilitation of many diseases, including hypertension, diabetes, hyperlipidemia, hyperuricemia, sleep disorder, cervical spondylosis, lumbar spondylosis, anxiety, depression and so on. Chinese Health Qigong Association suggests popularizing Baduanjin in communities to improve blood pressure, clinical symptoms and quality of life of patients with hypertension, which is beneficial to improving the activity tolerance of patients with heart disease.

IV Wuqinxi

Wuqinxi is an important traditional technique for daoyin and health preservation in China, which was created by Hua Tuo (about 145–208), a doctor in the Three Kingdoms period. Wuqinxi, a fitness exercise, mimics the activities of five animals, namely the tiger, deer, bear, ape and bird (crane), and has a good effect on the body and five zang viscera, which is widely spread. According to the *Book of Later Han Dynasty–Biography of Fang Shu–Biography of Hua Tuo*, "I have a skill, which is called Wuqinxi: the tiger, deer, bear, ape, and bird. It is also used as daoyin to eliminate diseases and benefit hoofs and feet. If you are uncomfortable, you can mimic the activities of an animal, and you will be happy and sweat. Thus, the complexion is rosy. Moreover, your body is light and you want to eat. If you keep practicing it, you will have smart eyes and ears and strong and intact teeth even at the age of 90." Among Hua Tuo's disciples, the famous ones are Wu Pu, Fan E, Li Dangzhi and others. Among them, Wu Pu is the author of *Wu Pu Materia Medica*. It is said that he practiced Wuqinxi and lived to be over 100 years old. In modern times, Wuqinxi is also widely used in the treatment of chronic diseases, such as endocrine and metabolic diseases and bone and joint diseases.

V Qigong

Qigong is also a traditional Chinese method of health care, health preservation and disease elimination. It is a physical and mental exercise to regulate the functions of meridians and zang-fu organs and promote the movement of qi and blood by means of adjusting breathing, physical activities and consciousness (breath, body and heart regulation) through rhythmic movements, exhalation and inhalation, and meditation, achieving the goal of strengthening the body, preventing and curing diseases, and prolonging life span. Qigong has been widely used in chronic diseases such as hypertension, coronary heart disease, insomnia, cerebral infarction and bone and joint diseases.

VI Moxa-wool moxibustion

Moxibustion, called "Jiuruo" and "Aijiu (moxa-wool moxibustion)" in ancient times, uses moxibustion cone or moxibustion grass to burn, fumigate and iron specific meridians and acupoints on the body surface, and stimulates the acupoints by means of the warmth of the fire. It has the effects of warming the channel for dispelling cold, supporting yang for relieving desertion, eliminating blood stasis and resolving hard mass, etc., and achieves the purpose of preventing and treating diseases. Moxibustion grass is most commonly used in clinic, so it is also called moxa-wool moxibustion. There are other methods, such as medicine-separated moxibustion, wicker moxibustion, common rush moxibustion and mulberry branch moxibustion. Nowadays, moxa stick moxibustion is still used most clinically.

Moxa-wool moxibustion is widely used in clinical cold pain of bone and joint diseases, including knee pain, knee osteoarthritis, cervical spondylosis, lumbar spondylosis, scapulohumeral periarthritis and so on. Moxa-wool moxibustion can also be used for some internal diseases, including chronic diarrhea, chronic cold

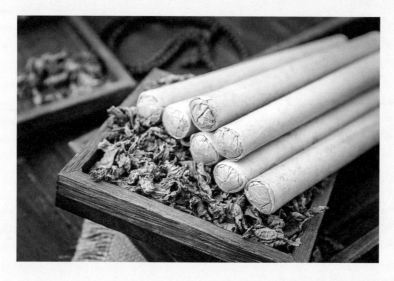

Moxa

abdominal pain, cold dysmenorrhea and so on. In addition, moxibustion has a certain effect of warmly invigorating yang qi, which can be used to regulate yang deficiency constitution.

VII Cupping

Cupping takes a cup as a tool, and mainly uses the methods of burning fire and pumping air to empty the air in the cup to form a negative pressure. Then, the cup can be adsorbed on the surface of the corresponding acupoints and specific parts, so that the local skin congestion and blood stasis can achieve the purpose of activating collateral, activating qi and promoting blood circulation, removing edema and relieving pain, and dispelling pathogenic wind and dispelling cold. Cupping therapy has a long history in ancient times. As early as *Prescriptions for Fifty-two Diseases*, there were records about the "Jiao method" (similar to the later cupping therapy). Cupping can be divided into fire cupping, water cupping and suction cupping. Nowadays, cupping therapy is widely used to treat rheumatism, shoulder and back pain, asthma, stomachache, abdominal pain, diarrhea, dysmenorrhea, acne, urticaria, facial paralysis and other diseases.

VIII Scraping

Scraping is one of the traditional Chinese medicine therapies, which is based on the TCM skin theory. It scrapes the relevant parts of the skin with horn, jade, fire cup and other instruments to dredge meridians and promote blood circulation for removing blood stasis. Scraping can be used to treat cervical spondylosis, suffering cold pathogen, heatstroke, suffering wind pathogen, gastrointestinal diseases, shoulder and back pain, skin diseases and so on.

IX Massage

Massage is also a traditional TCM therapy, which refers to the comprehensive use of pushing, holding, lifting, pinching, kneading and other techniques on the human body according to meridians and acupoints to achieve the purposes of dredging meridians, harmonizing qi and blood, dredging collaterals and relieving pain, eliminating pathogen and strengthening vital qi, harmonizing yin and yang and prolonging life. Its origin can be traced back to the ancient times, also known as rubbing, pressing correction and massage. It is clearly pointed out in the *Plain Questions–Dicussion on Appropriate Treating Methods Selection* that "in the central place, the terrain is flat and humid, and the products are abundant. Therefore, people have many kinds of food and their life is relatively comfortable. The diseases that occur here are mostly flaccidity, cold limbs, cold and heat. The treatment of these diseases should be daoyin and pressing correction. Therefore, the treatment of daoyin and pressing correction is promoted from the central region". It is also pointed out in the *Plain Questions–Blood, Qi, Physique and Will* that "for people who are physically comfortable but mentally depressed, the disease often occurs in the meridians, and acupuncture should be used for treatment. For people who are physically comfortable and mentally happy, the disease mostly occurs in the muscles, and acupuncture or stone needle should be used for treatment. For people who are physically hardworking but mentally happy, the disease often occurs in the tendons, hot ironing or daoyin should be used for treatment. For people who are physically and mentally distressed, the disease mostly occurs in the throat, and medicines should be used for treatment. For people who are often frightened, the meridians are obstructed due to the disorder of qi movement, and the disease is mostly numbness. Massage and medicinal wine should be used for treatment".

Nowadays, massage is commonly used in the treatment of tendon and bone diseases, including lumbar disc herniation, scapulohumeral periarthritis, low back pain and cervical spondylosis. In addition, some pediatric diseases, such as food accumulation, abdominal pain, diarrhea, fever, cough, etc., can also be treated with massage.

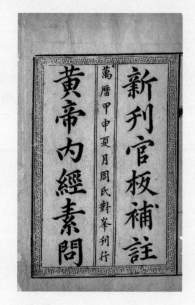

The Yellow Emperor's Inner Classic Basic Questions
(Huáng Dì Nèi Jīng Sù Wèn, 黄帝内经素问)

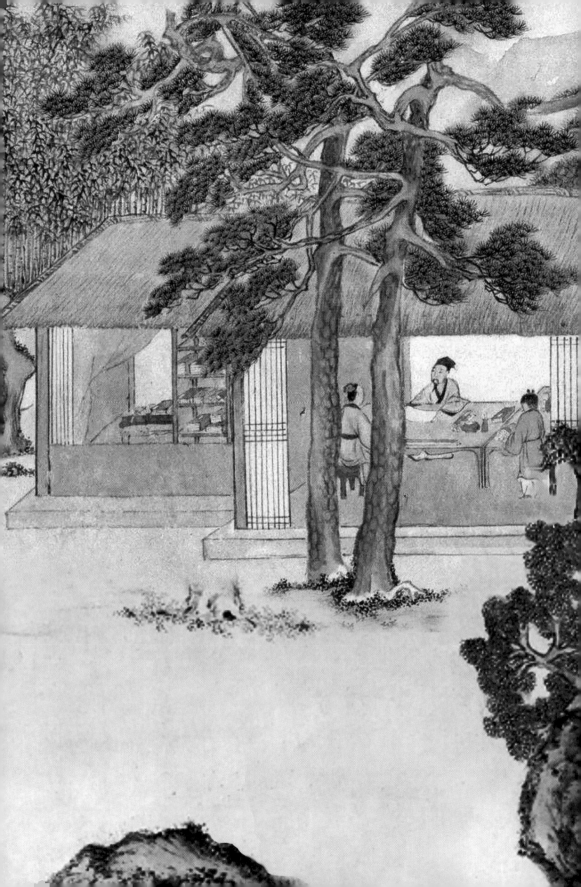

Chapter 2

The Wisdom of TCM Diagnosis and

Treatment of Common Diseases

Section 1
Respiratory System Diseases

Ⅰ Overview of respiratory system diseases

Cough, expectoration, asthma... I believe that almost everyone has had similar experiences, and doctors will tell them that "their lungs are bad" or "they have a cold". In fact, these are common symptoms of respiratory diseases. Respiratory diseases, as a common and frequently-occurring disease, are mainly located in the trachea, bronchus, lungs, and chest cavity. The mild cases are characterized by cough, expectoration, chest pain, and laborious breathing, and the severe cases lead to dyspnea, hypoxia, and even death. Common respiratory diseases include acute upper respiratory tract infection, pneumonia, chronic obstructive pulmonary disease (COPD), bronchial asthma, pulmonary nodules, and so on.

In clinical treatment, therapeutic medicines include antibiotics, bronchodilators, sputum thinners, antiallergic medicines, and so on. However, we have found that there are still many children with repeated upper respiratory tract infections due to poor resistance; elderly patients are insensitive to antibiotics and have a poor curative effect on pneumonia. COPD recurs after they get a cold; children with bronchial asthma must carry with them antispasmolytics, such as tiotropium bromide (Spiriva) and salmeterol fluticasone (Seretide); patients with pulmonary nodules less than 1 cm can only be reexamined regularly, instead of receiving any intervention.

In recent years, the clinical value of TCM in treating respiratory diseases has been increasingly recognized internationally. Especially in the prevention and treatment of corona virus disease 2019 (COVID-19), the curative effect of Chinese medicine in reducing fever and shortening the course of fever has been valued and recognized. In fact, TCM has a unique cognitive system and therapeutic prescription for respiratory diseases. Respiratory diseases belong to the categories of "cough", "cold", "wheezing", "dyspnea syndrome", "lung distension", etc. in TCM. Their disease location is mainly in the lung. The primary pathogenesis is the lung qi failing in dispersing and descending, and the disorder of lung qi, which is closely related to all zang-fu viscera of the whole body. Studies have found that TCM has shown a certain value in quickly reducing fever, relieving cough and expectoration symptoms, reducing the frequency of COPD and bronchial asthma, and improving the quality of life. This section will focus on the clinical understanding and treatment of TCM in the acute upper respiratory tract infection, bronchial asthma, pulmonary nodules, COPD, and influenza.

|| Treatises on respiratory system diseases

1 Acute upper respiratory tract infection

Acute upper respiratory tract infection, commonly known as cold, is a general term including acute inflammation of the nasal cavity, pharynx, or throat. In terms of clinical symptoms, the common clinical manifestations of this disease include sneezing, stuffy nose, runny nose, cough, expectoration, pharyngeal discomfort, tears, fever, aversion to cold, fatigue, headache, poor breathing, hoarseness, swelling and pain of submandibular lymph nodes, etc.

In clinical diagnosis, in addition to discomfort symptoms, it is necessary to combine the course of the disease, blood routine, and bacterial and viral culture results to make a precise diagnosis and guide rational medicine use.

In clinical treatment, besides symptomatic treatment, antibiotics, commonly known as anti-inflammatory medicines, are the most frequently used and most known to ordinary people. For some people, antibiotics can cure diseases, but only in the right dose and type at the right time. Unfortunately, a large amount of long-term use of antibiotics is prone to drug resistance and related adverse reactions, including intestinal flora imbalance and antibiotic-related diarrhea, which affect the clinical efficacy to a certain extent.

In fact, in the early stage of this disease, many patients will choose to take Chinese medicinals. If the treatment is timely, it is likely to block the progress of the disease quickly. Finally, the disease will be cured. According to TCM, acute upper respiratory tract infection belongs to the category of "cold", and its etiology is mainly exogenous or combined with deficiency of vital qi.

In clinical treatment, Xiaochaihu Granule and Ganmao Qingre Granule are commonly used. Xiaochaihu Decoction, a classic prescription, comes from the

Treatise on Cold Pathogenic Diseases. It is composed of 7 Chinese medicinals, such as Chaihu (Bupleuri Radix), Huangqin (Scutellariae Radix), Banxia (Pinelliae Rhizoma), Shengjiang (Zingiberis Rhizoma Recens), Renshen (Ginseng Radix et Rhizoma), Dazao (Jujubae Fructus) and Gancao (Glycyrrhizae Radix et Rhizoma). It has the effect of reconciling Shaoyang. In ancient times, Xiaochaihu Decoction was mainly used to treat cold pathogenic diseases and Shaoyang syndrome. In patients with upper respiratory tract infection, if fever is accompanied by vomiting, a bitter taste, dry mouth, sore throat, and loss of appetite, this is the typical indication for us to use Xiaochaihu Granule. It is worth noting that in the north, many people will "get on their throats" immediately after suffering cold pathogen, and they will immediately say that their throats are uncomfortable. Patients will say that they are getting inflamed. This is the indication of Xiaochaihu Decoction/Granule in TCM. We recommend that patients take it orally, 1–2 bags each time, 3 times daily.

Ganmao Qingre Granule is a prescription developed by later doctors. It is composed of 11 Chinese medicinals, including Jingjiesui (Schizonepetae Spica), Bohe (Menthae Haplocalycis Herba), Fangfeng (Saposhnikoviae Radix), Chaihu (Bupleuri Radix), Zisuye (Perillae Folium), Gegen (Puerariae Lobatae Radix), Jiegeng (Platycodonis Radix), Kuxinren (Armeniacae Semen Amarum), Baizhi (Angelicae Dahuricae Radix), Kudiding (Corydalis Bungeanae Herba) and Lugen (Phragmitis Rhizoma). This prescription has the effects of relieving exterior with pungent and warm-natured medicines, and relieving exterior and clearing heat. It can treat cold with wind-cold combined with depression transforming into heat. Unlike Xiaochaihu Granule, which is mainly used for bitter mouth, dry throat, and sore throat, Ganmao Qingre Granule can be used when patients have both headache and fever, aversion to cold, body pain, thin nasal discharge and cough, and endogenous heat symptoms, such as dry throat and yellow urine. The routine method is to take them with boiled water, 1 bag each time, twice daily.

2 Bronchial asthma

In our daily life, we often see some people who go everywhere with a bottle of throat spray in their pockets, and these people suffer from what is commonly known as "asthma".

The scientific name of this "asthma" is bronchial asthma, a chronic inflammatory disease of the airway involving various cells such as eosinophils and mast cells. Its typical symptoms are paroxysmal dyspnea, mainly exhalation, even forced sitting, often accompanied by wheezing, cough, expectoration, chest oppression, cyanotic lips, etc. Some patients only present with cough, called cough variant asthma; some patients, especially teenagers, whose onset is with chest oppression, cough, and difficulty breathing during exercising, called exercise asthma.

The causes of the disease include dust mites, pollen, inhalation of cold air, medicines, and some foods. The disease can occur within minutes and last from hours to days.

In clinical diagnosis, in addition to typical clinical symptoms, such as dyspnea and wheezing rale, diagnosis can only be confirmed by combining with the disease history, blood routine, allergen determination, chest X-ray, lung function determination, and blood gas analysis and other specialized examination results.

In clinical treatment, the well-known medicines include antispasmolytic drug—budesonide formoterol, salmeterol fluticasone (Seretide), and so on. However, some patients may have increased blood sugar, osteoporosis, decreased immunity, drug tolerance, decreased curative effect, and many other reactions after taking the drug. There are also some patients who suffer from repeated attacks of bronchial asthma, which can be relieved after medication and relapse after drug withdrawal, so they come to the clinic to seek TCM treatment. TCM has certain clinical advantages in relieving dyspnea symptoms, reducing attack frequency, and stopping and reducing Western medicine during bronchial asthma attacks.

In TCM, bronchial asthma belongs to the category of "wheezing". Etiology includes exogenous pathogen invasion, improper diet, weakness after illness, emotional change, overstrain and family congenital endowment. In pathogenesis, this disease is related to retained phlegm lodging in the lung and deficiency of vital qi.

In clinical treatment, it is necessary to distinguish whether bronchial asthma belongs to acute exacerbation or remission. Shegan Mahuang Decoction is a commonly used classic prescription for those in the acute exacerbation stage with frequent onset and severe symptoms in a short time. Shegan Mahuang Decoction comes from the *Synopsis of Golden Chamber*. It is composed of 9 Chinese medicinals, such as Shegan (Belamcandae Rhizoma), Mahuang (Ephedrae Herba), Shengjiang (Zingiberis Rhizoma Recens), Xixin (Asari Radix et Rhizoma), Ziwan (Asteris Radix et Rhizoma), Kuandonghua (Farfarae Flos), Wuweizi (Schisandrae Chinensis Fructus), Dazao (Jujubae Fructus) and Banxia (Pinelliae Rhizoma). It can warm lung for dispelling cold, and dissipate phlegm and relieve panting. This prescription is suitable for patients with asthma accompanied by tachypnea, wheezing in the throat, chest oppression, slight cough, a small amount of white sticky phlegm, no thirst in the mouth, or thirst with a desire for hot drinks, onset in cold weather, or aversion to cold, sneezing, and runny nose. Modern clinical studies have shown that Shegan Mahuang Decoction can reduce airway hyperreactivity.

In the remission period of bronchial asthma, Chinese patent medicine—Yupingfeng Granule, is commonly used in strengthening constitution, improving lung function, and reducing attack frequency. Yupingfeng Granule comes from *Effective Formulae Handed Down for Generations*, which is composed of Huangqi (Astragali Radix), Fangfeng (Saposhnikoviae Radix), and Baizhu (Atractylodis Macrocephalae Rhizoma). They have the effects of benefiting qi, consolidating the exterior, and arresting sweating. In this period, if a patient has shortness of breath, aggravation after activities, fear of wind, sweating all day long, vulnerability to cold in windy weather, or a slight wheezing sound in the throat and expectoration with clear and white sputum, he/she can take Yupingfeng Granule orally to strengthen the constitution. Take 5 g each time, and 3 times daily.

References

LIN C C, WANG Y Y, CHEN S M, et al. Shegan-Mahuang Decoction ameliorates asthmatic airway hyperresponsiveness by downregulating Th2/Th17 cells but upregulating CD4[+] FoxP3 + Tregs. Journal of Ethnopharmacology, 2020, 253: e112656.

3 Pulmonary nodules

Many people have no discomfort at ordinary times, and they are in good health. A chest X-ray shows that there is a nodule in their lungs on a routine physical examination. Thus, they are scared and overwhelmed, thinking they have an incurable disease. Medically speaking, pulmonary nodules refer to focal round dense shadows with various sizes, clear or fuzzy edges, and diameters less than or equal to 3 cm on lung images.

In the cause of the disease, the formation of pulmonary nodules may be related to smoking, air pollution, inhalation of industrial dust particles and sequelae of pulmonary diseases. Pulmonary nodules can be malignant, but not all nodules are "sick", and not all pulmonary nodules need treatment. Therefore, when nodules are found in the lungs, do not panic. Actively seek the help of professional doctors and follow their advice.

In addition to imaging results, the differential diagnosis of benign and malignant pulmonary nodules should be combined with the patient's clinical symptoms, medical history, occupational characteristics, living habits, as well as blood routine, sputum culture, tuberculosis bacilli, tumor markers and other test results, especially the puncture results of pulmonary nodules. Only after careful evaluation can the final diagnosis be made.

In the population with pulmonary nodules, when the diameter is less than 1 cm, and there is no discomfort; moreover, the results of blood drawing and sputum culture are normal, these patients can be observed for 3 months before reexamination. If the nodule does not continue to grow, it can be reviewed regularly. If the nodule is found to be significantly enlarged, pathological tissue should be obtained by puncture for biopsy, and the following treatment plan should be determined according to the pathological results.

In clinical treatment, many patients are unwilling to wait passively, but hope for TCM therapy. By improving their lifestyle combined with internal administration of Chinese medicinals to soften and resolve hard mass and dissipate phlegm and promote blood circulation, they hope to achieve the purpose of reducing the nodules in the reexamination after 3 months.

In TCM, according to its clinical symptoms, pulmonary nodules can be classified as "cough", "asthmatic syndrome", "lung tuberculosis", "lung cancer", and other categories. In pathogenesis, pulmonary nodules belong to the tangible pathogen, mainly related to qi stagnation, internal stagnation of phlegm-turbidity, and static blood, and blocked meridians. According to the clinical experience of TCM, Xiaochaihu Decoction and Xiaoluo Pill are commonly used, although there is still a lack of evidence-based support.

Xiaochaihu Decoction comes from *Treatise on Cold Pathogenic Diseases*, which is composed of 7 Chinese medicinals: Chaihu (Bupleuri Radix), Huangqin (Radix Scutellariae), Banxia (Pinelliae Rhizoma), Shengjiang (Zingiberis Rhizoma Recens), Renshen (Ginseng Radix et Rhizoma), Dazao (Jujubae Fructus) and Gancao (Glycyrrhizae Radix et Rhizoma). It has the effect of reconciling Shaoyang. We have found that many patients with pulmonary nodules have certain factors of stagnation of liver qi and qi, such as chest tightness and dysphoria, loss of appetite, nausea, and vomiting, dry mouth and a bitter taste, dizziness, and so on. The prescription can be based on Xiaochaihu Decoction and gets modified with symptoms.

Xiaoluo Pill comes from *Medical Revelations* written by Cheng Zhongling, a doctor in the Qing Dynasty. This prescription is composed of Zhebeimu (Fritillariae Thunbergii Bulbus), Xuanshen (Scrophulariae Radix), and Muli (Ostreae Concha). It has the effects of resolving phlegm with clear-moistening medicines, and softening and resolving hard masses. TCM believes that pulmonary nodules are related to the blockade of phlegm-turbidity. This prescription is suitable for patients with pulmonary nodules accompanied by cough and expectoration with yellow sticky and thick sputum, chest oppression, shortness of breath, thirst with a desire for cold drinks, red tongue with yellow fur.

4 Chronic obstructive pulmonary disease

We often see such patients who look like they have a cylindrical chest, like a bucket, and seem to be holding a breath all the time, panting and coughing when they walk a little faster. They breathe shallowly and fast in the usual quiet state, gasping for breath, coughing with sputum from time to time. Most of these people have chronic obstructive pulmonary disease (COPD for short).

COPD is chronic bronchitis or emphysema characterized by airflow obstruction. Chronic bronchitis refers to cough and expectoration for more than 3 months every year and for 2 or more consecutive years after excluding other diseases with cough, expectoration, and wheezing symptoms. Emphysema refers to an abnormally prolonged distension of the distal bronchioles of the end lung with the destruction of bronchioles and alveoli without significant pulmonary fibrosis. COPD can be diagnosed when lung function tests of patients with chronic bronchitis and emphysema indicate persistent airflow restriction.

In etiology, this disease is related to smoking, long-term exposure to high-concentration occupational dust, repeated respiratory tract infection, old age, immune dysfunction, and many other factors. Clinical symptoms include chronic cough, expectoration, gasping, and chest oppression. In clinical diagnosis, in addition to the above symptoms, the patient can be seen with an enlarged anterior-posterior thoracic diameter during physical examination and a "barrel-shaped chest". The diagnosis can be made by combining the medical history, living habits and environment with the results of auxiliary examinations (chest radiograph, lung CT, etc., especially lung function examination).

In clinical treatment, symptomatic treatment is applied with commonly used medicines, such as salmeterol fluticasone (Seretide), tiotropium bromide (Spiriva), salbutamol sulfate (Ventolin), diprophylline, etc., can be said to be "old friends" of patients with COPD. These medicines are quick to take effect, easy to carry, and can effectively relieve symptoms during an attack. However, there are still some people who will have gastrointestinal discomfort, palpitation, medicine allergy, and other side effects after use. A poor curative effect and repeated attacks will affect their quality of life.

TCM in the treatment of COPD can relieve clinical symptoms, reduce the frequency of attacks, and at the same time, enhance the patient's constitution. In TCM, COPD belongs to the category of "lung distension". In terms of etiology, externally-contracted pathogens can lead to its onset or aggravation. In pathogenesis, lung deficiency and phlegm-turbidity retention due to long-term sickness lead to the distension and fullness of lung qi and loss of astringency and descent. The primary symptoms are chest tightness like blocking, gasping and qi ascending, and cough with excessive phlegm.

In clinical treatment, Xiaoqinglong Decoction and Shegan Mahuang Decoction are commonly used. Xiaoqinglong Decoction comes from the *Treatise on Cold Pathogenic Diseases*, which is composed of 8 Chinese medicinals: Mahuang (Ephedrae Herba),

Guizhi (Cinnamomi Ramulus), Baishao (Paeoniae Radix Alba), Gancao (Glycyrrhizae Radix et Rhizoma), Ganjiang (Zingiberis Rhizoma), Xixin (Asari Radix et Rhizoma), Banxia (Pinelliae Rhizoma) and Wuweizi (Schisandrae Chinensis Fructus). It has the effects of relieving superficies and dispelling cold, and warming the lung for resolving fluid retention. The original text says: "The patient coughs with asthma. Especially, when the patient has asthma, he must rely on some thing to breathe, instead of being supine, and Xiaoqinglong Decoction can be used." "The patient suffers from cold pathogenic diseases and has water pathogen in the stomach. He coughs and pants mildly. He also has a fever, but is not thirsty." Patients with COPD have severe cough, asthma, inability to lie flat, foam-like thin white sputum, fear of cold, soreness all over, and do not want to drink water or desire for warm water after suffering cold pathogen. They can choose Xiaoqinglong Decoction. Decoct with water, or take Chinese medicinal formula granules with boiled water, one dose daily, and once in the morning and once in the afternoon.

Shegan Mahuang Decoction comes from *Synopsis of Golden Chamber*, and its indication is recorded in the original text as "cough with upper reversal of qi, a frog's voice in the throat". The prescription is composed of 9 Chinese medicinals: Shegan (Belamcandae Rhizoma), Mahuang (Ephedrae Herba), Shengjiang (Zingiberis Rhizoma Recens), Xixin (Asari Radix et Rhizoma), Ziwan (Asteris Radix et Rhizoma), Kuandonghua (Farfarae Flos), Wuweizi (Schisandrae Chinensis Fructus), Dazao (Jujubae Fructus) and Banxia (Pinelliae Rhizoma). It has the effects of warming the lung for dispelling cold, and dissipating phlegm and relieving panting. This prescription is suitable for patients with acute exacerbation of COPD, such as tachypnea, wheezing in the throat, chest oppression, slight cough, coughing with a small amount of white sticky phlegm, no thirst, or thirst with a liking for hot drinks, fear of cold, or aversion to cold, sneezing, and runny nose. Cold weather or any cold stimulus leads to its onset. Decoct Chinese medicinal pieces with water, or take Chinese medicinal formula granules with boiled water, one dose daily and once in the morning and once in the afternoon.

References

KAO S T, WANG S T, YU C K, et al. The effect of Chinese herbal medicine, xiao-qing-long tang (XQLT), on allergen-induced bronchial inflammation in mite-sensitized mice[J]. Allergy, 2000, 55(12): 1127-1133.

5 Influenza A

Although it has been 10 years since the outbreak of influenza A (H1N1), it is still hard to forget. Influenza A, commonly known as "H1N1", is an acute respiratory infectious disease caused by the influenza A virus. H refers to hemagglutinin and N to neuraminidase of influenza A virus, respectively. There are 15 kinds of H and 9 kinds of N, and the so-called H1N1 is one subtype of influenza A virus.

Influenza A mainly spreads through contact and airborne droplets. It frequently occurs in winter and spring in the north, and can be prevalent all year round in the south. The early symptoms of human infection with influenza A are similar to those of the common cold. The difference is that influenza A has an acute onset, apparent epidemic and outbreak, apparent poisoning symptoms, such as fear of cold, high fever, headache and whole body muscle soreness, mild nasopharyngeal symptoms, conjunctivitis, diarrhea or vomiting, loss of appetite, etc. In severe cases, severe pneumonia may be complicated, and even death may occur due to shock and respiratory failure.

In clinical diagnosis, in addition to the pathogenesis and clinical symptoms, it is necessary to combine blood routine examination, pathogenic examination of nasopharynx, lower respiratory tract secretion or oral gargle, with the detection results of serum viral antigen and antibody before a precise diagnosis can be made.

In clinical treatment, suspected and confirmed patients should be isolated first. Symptomatic and supportive treatment should be carried out based on the routine application of antiviral medicines, such as oseltamivir and paramivir. Besides virus virulence, autoimmune status is an essential factor in determining prognosis. Uncomplicated influenza A generally has a good prognosis. At the same time, elderly and frail patients are prone to complications such as pneumonia, toxemia, which are easy to progress to severe cases, and often secondary infection during treatment.

TCM has apparent advantages in reducing fever quickly, cutting off the disease course, strengthening patients' constitution, and reducing severe cases. In TCM, influenza A belongs to the category of "influenza". In etiology, it is induced by exposure to seasonal virus. In pathogenesis, it is mainly related to pathogen invading the lung-defense phase and disharmony of defensive exterior.

In clinical treatment, Yinqiao Powder and Maxing Shigan Decoction are commonly used. Yinqiao Powder comes from *Detailed Analysis of Epidemic Warm Diseases* written by Wu Jutong, a doctor in the Qing Dynasty. It is composed of 10 Chinese medicinals, including Lianqiao (Forsythiae Fructus), Jinyinhua (Lonicerae Japonicae Flos), Jiegeng (Platycodonis Radix), Bohe (Menthae Haplocalycis Herba), Zhuye (Lophatheri Herba), Gancao (Glycyrrhizae Radix et Rhizoma), Jingjie (Schizonepetae Herba), Dandouchi (Sojae Semen Praeparatum), Niubangzi (Arctii Fructus) and Lugen (Phragmitis Rhizoma). It has the effects of resolving superficies syndrome with pungent and cool-natured medicinals, and clearing heat and removing toxicity. Yinqiao Powder can be used when patients with influenza A present such symptoms as high fever, slight aversion to wind and cold, no sweat or sweating and unsmooth sweat, headache, sore throat, cough, thirst, and red tongue tip, etc.

Maxing Shigan Decoction comes from the *Treatise on Cold Pathogenic Diseases* written by Zhang Zhongjing, a medical sage. It is composed of Mahuang (Ephedrae Herba), Xingren (Armeniacae Semen Amarum), Shigao (Gypsum Fibrosum), and Gancao (Glycyrrhizae Radix et Rhizoma). It has the effects of resolving exterior syndrome with pungent and cool-natured medicinals, and clearing lung heat and relieving panting. It is suitable for patients with influenza A with persistent fever, cough, and acute dyspnea, flapping of nasal wings, thirst, sweat, or no sweat. Clinically, Yinqiao Powder and Maxing Shigan Decoction are often used in combination. A randomized, controlled, and clinical study of Yinqiao Powder combined with Maxing Shigan Decoction in treating influenza A, led by Academician Wang Chen of Peking Union Medical College, included 410 patients, found that compared with oseltamivir alone, the intervention of Yinqiao Powder combined with Maxing Shigan Decoction for 5 days could significantly shorten the duration of fever. In the way of taking it, Chinese medicinal pieces are usually decocted with water, 1 dose daily, and once in the morning and once in the afternoon.

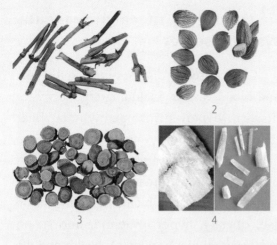

Maxing Shigan Decoction
1. Mahuang; 2. Kuxingren;
3. Gancao; 4. Shigao.

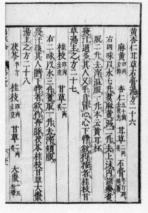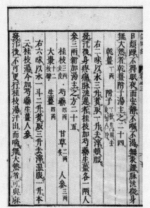

Articles of Maxing Shigan Decoction

References

WANG C, CAO B, LIU Q Q, et al. Oseltamivir compared with the Chinese traditional therapy maxingshigan-yinqiaosan in the treatment of H1N1 influenza: a randomized trial[J]. Ann Intern Med, 2011,155(4):217-225.

Section 2
Cardiovascular System Diseases

I Overview of cardiovascular system diseases

Cardiovascular diseases involve the heart and blood vessels, including coronary heart disease, hypertension, arrhythmia, heart failure, myocarditis, valvular heart disease, cardiomyopathy, and so on. The occurrence of cardiovascular diseases is closely related to many risk factors, including hypertension, smoking, diabetes, lack of exercise, obesity, hyperlipidemia, and so on. Cardiovascular diseases have become a severe threat to people's health and life, with high mortality and disability rates.

In the past 30 years, modern medicine has made significant progress in the primary and secondary prevention of cardiovascular diseases, including secondary prevention for coronary heart disease, interventional therapy, and coronary artery bypass grafting; 5 kinds of antihypertensive medicines for hypertension, research and development of new antihypertensive medicines and percutaneous renal artery sympathetic ablation; ezetimibe and PCSK9 inhibitors for hyperlipidemia; and new medicines for heart failure, such as shakubactril valsartan sodium tablets and levosimendan. However, the mortality, morbidity, and prevalence of cardiovascular diseases (mainly coronary heart disease, stroke, etc.) are on the rise in China. At present, the mortality rate of cardiovascular disease in China ranks first among all diseases, accounting for about 2 out of every 5 deaths. In addition, in health economics, since 1980, the number of patients discharged from hospitals and medical expenses of patients with cardiovascular and cerebrovascular diseases in China has been increasing continuously, and increased rapidly after 2000. Cardiovascular disease has become a major global public health problem.

However, we have found that the side effects and intolerance caused by combined therapy greatly limited the clinical efficacy. In particular, some elderly patients have aspirin resistance, clopidogrel resistance, secondary nitroglycerin failure, diuretic resistance, liver function increase and myalgia caused by statins, headache caused by isosorbide mononitrate, sexual function decline caused by antihypertensive medicines, etc., which seriously plague the majority of patients. At the same time, clinically, we also found that in some people, the use of TCM can benefit some patients with cardiovascular diseases, which can not only improve clinical symptoms, reduce the frequency of attacks and alleviate adverse reactions, but even some patients can achieve the goal of stopping and reducing the dosage of Western medicine (under the guidance of doctors). Therefore, here, we will focus on the TCM clinical treatment scheme and methods for coronary heart disease, hypertension, arrhythmia, heart failure, viral myocarditis and cardiomyopathy.

‖ Treatises on cardiovascular system diseases

1 Coronary heart disease

Coronary heart disease is a heart disease caused by atherosclerosis of the coronary artery, which leads to stenosis or occlusion of the vascular lumen and myocardial ischemia, hypoxia, or necrosis. The World Health Organization (WHO) divides coronary heart disease into 5 categories: asymptomatic myocardial ischemia, angina pectoris, myocardial infarction, ischemic heart failure (ischemic heart disease), and sudden death.

Regarding clinical symptoms, the primary manifestations are increased pain in the precordia after physical activity and emotional excitement, mainly colic, squeezing pain, and feeling of chest oppression. Chest pain can be radiated to the left shoulder, arm, and even the little finger and ring finger, and can also be radiated to the neck, jaw, teeth, abdomen, etc. Symptoms can be relieved by rest or by nitroglycerin. However, some patients have atypical symptoms, only showing precordial discomfort, palpitation or fatigue, or gastrointestinal symptoms, and even some diabetic patients have no discomfort.

In clinical diagnosis, it is necessary to combine clinical symptoms and auxiliary examination to find evidence of myocardial ischemia or coronary artery occlusion, as well as markers of myocardial injury. The most commonly used examination methods include electrocardiogram, treadmill exercise test, radionuclide myocardial imaging, coronary angiography, and so on.

In Western medical treatment, smoking cessation and alcohol restriction, low-fat and low-salt diet, proper physical exercise, weight control, and other changes in living habits are included; antiplatelet, anticoagulation, beta-blockers, nitrates, statins, and other medical therapies are included; interventional therapy (endovascular balloon dilatation and stent implantation), surgical coronary artery bypass grafting, etc., are included.

Although Western medicine has made significant progress in diagnosis and treatment, there are still some patients with chest pain and oppression that are not relieved. Some patients have aspirin resistance, headache caused by intolerance of nitrate medicines, muscle pain caused by intolerance of statins, and other problems. Some patients will actively seek TCM treatment, which is especially common among elderly patients.

In TCM, coronary heart disease belongs to the category of "heart pain". In terms of etiology, the occurrence of this disease is mainly related to many factors, such as internal invasion of cold pathogen, eating disorder, emotional disorder, overstrain and internal damage, old age, physical weakness, etc. In pathogenesis, there are 2 situations: deficiency and excess. Deficiency syndrome is mainly due to malnutrition of the heart vessel and deficiency-induced pain, while excess syndrome is due to blockade of the heart vessel and stoppage-induced pain.

In modern clinical practice, the classic prescription Gualou Xiebai Banxia Decoction and a Chinese patent medicine Shexiang Baoxin Pill are especially widely used. Gualou Xiebai Banxia Decoction comes from the *Synopsis of Golden Chamber* written by Zhang Zhongjing. It is composed of Gualou (Trichosanthis Fructus), Xiebai (Allii Macrostemonis Bulbus), and Jiangbanxia (Pinelliae Rhizoma Praeparatum cum Zingibere et Alumine), which can dredge yang and resolve hard mass, and broaden the chest. Although the ancients did not know what caused coronary heart disease, in the theory of TCM, it was because of phlegm-turbidity and pathogen qi blocking meridians, which led to chest yang obstruction. This understanding is similar to that of the pathological mechanism of coronary heart disease in Western medicine. Modern pharmacological studies have also found that this prescription has the functions of protecting myocardial cells, improving cardiac function, lowering lipids, and relieving atherosclerosis.

Shexiang Baoxin Pill, a Chinese patent medicine, was developed by Professor

Dai Ruihong, Department of Cardiology, Huashan Hospital Affiliated to Fudan University. Based on Suhexiang Pill, a classic prescription in the Song Dynasty, the effective ingredients were screened and developed one by one by using modern pharmacological research methods. The patent emdicine has the effects of warmly dredging with aromatic natured medicinals and benefiting qi, and strengthening the heart, and can be used for coronary heart disease caused by stagnation of qi and blood stasis. Up to now, Shexiang Baoxin Pill has been used clinically for nearly 40 years. In particular, the MUST research published in the *Chinese Medical Journal* in 2021 has attracted much attention, which confirms the clinical value of Shexiang Baoxin Pill. The study was led by Academician Ge Junbo, with the participation of 97 tertiary hospitals in 22 provinces, municipalities, and autonomous regions. A total of 2,673 patients with stable coronary heart disease were included and followed up for 2 years. Studies have shown that based on aspirin and statin therapy, compared with the placebo group, the risk of major adverse cardiovascular events (MACE) is reduced by 26.9 % after adding Shexiang Baoxin Pill. In addition, after 18 months of continuous medication, the K-M curve gradually separated, and the degree of separation gradually increased, showing long-term effectiveness and safety. Moreover, taking Shexiang Baoxin Pill for a long time can significantly improve the stability and frequency score of angina pectoris, which also indicates that Shexiang Baoxin Pill can effectively relieve the clinical symptoms of patients with coronary heart disease and significantly improve the quality of life. These pills taste bitter, pungent and cool, with a feeling of tongue numbness, and they are dark brown shiny water pills. Their broken sections are brown and yellow. Take 2 pills each time, 3 times daily; or when angina pectoris symptoms occur, take them.

References

GE J B, FAN W H, ZHOU J M, et al. Efficacy and safety of Shexiang Baoxin pill (MUSKARDIA) in patients with stable coronary artery disease: a multicenter, double-blind, placebo-controlled phase IV randomized clinical trial[J]. Chin Med J (Engl), 2020, 134 (2): 185-192.

2 Hypertension

Hypertension refers to a group of clinical syndromes characterized by increased systemic arterial blood pressure (systolic blood pressure ≥ 140 mmHg and diastolic blood pressure ≥ 90 mmHg), possibly accompanied by functional or organic damage to vital target organs, such as the heart, brain, and kidney. Hypertension is the most common chronic disease in the clinic. It is also one of the most critical risk factors for cardiovascular and cerebrovascular diseases. With the increase of age, blood pressure gradually rises. There are 245 million patients with hypertension in China, which has become a major public health problem.

In terms of clinical symptoms, the symptoms of hypertension vary from person to person, and there is no discomfort in the early stage. Many young patients only find that their blood pressure rises during physical examination. Common clinical symptoms include dizziness, headache, stiff neck, fatigue, palpitation, inattention, memory loss, limb numbness, and so on. The above discomfort will be aggravated after fatigue, mental stress, and emotional fluctuations. The symptoms are relieved after rest.

In clinical diagnosis, the diagnosis can be made according to medical history, physical examination, and laboratory results. This disease is divided into primary and secondary hypertension, which needs to be differentiated. The causes of secondary hypertension include renal parenchymal disease, renal artery stenosis, primary aldosteronism, pheochromocytoma and so on.

In clinical treatment, the primary goal is to keep blood pressure up to standard, and the ultimate goal is to minimize the incidence and mortality of cardiovascular and cerebrovascular diseases. Treatment methods include lifestyle regulation and medication. Lifestyle regulation includes weight control, a low-salt and low-fat diet, calcium and potassium supplementation, exercise, smoking cessation, alcohol restriction, and mental stress reduction. 5 commonly used antihypertensive medicines include diuretics, beta-blockers, calcium channel blockers, angiotensin-converting enzyme inhibitors, and angiotensin II receptor blockers.

Although Western medicine has made significant progress in the medical treatment of hypertension, there are still "three highs", "three lows", and "three noes", and the prevention and treatment situation is still grim. Clinically, although the blood pressure of some patients is up to standard, dizziness, headache, and discomfort still exist. There are also some patients with decreased sexual function, soreness of the waist and knees, weakness of limbs, and decreased physical strength due to long-term medication and combined treatment, which seriously reduces medication compliance. Currently, the overall regulatory advantages of TCM in treating hypertension have been concerned by international authoritative magazines.

In TCM, hypertension belongs to the category of "headache" and "vertigo". In etiology, this disease is mainly related to the emotional disorders, eating disorders, overstrain, and internal damage, physical weakness due to long-term illness, etc. In pathogenesis, hypertension is related to deficiency of qi and blood and insufficiency of kidney essence, which leads to the emptiness of brain marrow and malnutrition of clear orifices, or upper hyperactivity of liver yang, the adverse rising of phlegm-fire, and static blood blocking orifices, which disturb clear orifices.

In modern clinical practice, the classic prescription Tianma Gouteng Decoction and Chinese patent medicine Songling Xuemaikang Capsule are incredibly widely used. Tianma Gouteng Decoction comes from the *New Meaning of Syndrome Treatment of Miscellaneous Diseases* by Hu Guangci, a modern doctor. The whole prescription is composed of Tianma (Gastrodiae Rhizoma), Gouteng (Uncariae Ramulus Cum Uncis), Shengjueming (raw Cassiae Semen), Zhizi (Gardeniae Fructus), Huangqin (Scutellariae Radix), Chuanniuxi (Cyathulae Radix), Sangjisheng (Taxilli Herba), Duzhong (Eucommiae Cortex), Shouwuteng (Polygoni Multiflori Caulis), Fushen (Sclerotium Poriae Pararadicis), and Yimucao (Leonuri Herba). This prescription has the effects of suppressing hyperactive liver for calming endogenous wind, clearing heat and promoting blood circulation, and nourishing the liver and kidney. It is mainly used for treating syndrome of hyperactivity of liver yang and upward disturbance of wind-yang. We have found that this prescription can be widely used in upper hyperactivity of liver yang syndrome of hypertension. It has a better effect on incipient hypertension and young hypertension patients with a short course of the disease or without antihypertensive medicine intervention. Moreover, it is also suitable for acute and severe diseases, such as grade 3 hypertension, hypertension crisis, and hypertension emergency. In 2020, a randomized, placebo-controlled clinical trial was published in *Circulation* by Professor Wang Jiguang of Shanghai Ruijin Hospital and his teram. A total of 251 patients with occult hypertension were included. Occult hypertension means that the blood pressure in the clinic is less than 140/90 mmHg. However, the systolic blood pressure is 135–150 mmHg or the diastolic blood pressure is 85–95 mmHg during ambulatory blood pressure monitoring. Studies have shown that 44.4 % of patients in Tianma Gouteng Granule group have daily time blood pressure drop of ≥ 10 / 5 mmHg. Tianma Gouteng, Granule a Chinese patent medicine, is effective for occult hypertension, and there is no adverse reaction during the treatment.

Chinese patent medicine Songling Xuemaikang Capsule is composed of fresh pine needles and Gegen (Puerariae Lobatae Radix) in a ratio of 6 : 1, and Zhenzhu (Margarita) layer powders are added as auxiliary materials, which has the effects of suppressing hyperactive liver and subsiding yang, and calming the heart for tranquillization. In 2022, *Cardiovascular Quality and Outcomes* published a randomized, double-blind, double-simulated, multicenter clinical study of Songling Xuemaikang Capsule in treating essential hypertension (grade 1) online. A total of 628 patients with grade 1 hypertension were included. The patients were randomly divided into the Songling Xuemaikang group and the control medicine group with a ratio of 1 : 1. The course of treatment was 8 weeks. The results showed that Songling Xuemaikang Capsule was not inferior to the control medicines in reducing diastolic blood pressure. In reducing systolic blood pressure and improving 24-hour ambulatory blood pressure, they are equally effective; in reducing serum total cholesterol and improving hypertension symptoms (especially the symptoms related to hyperactivity of liver yang), Songling Xuemaikang Capsule is significantly superior to the control medicines.

In addition, traditional sports, such as Tai Chi, Baduanjin, Qigong, and Yoga, acupuncture therapy, moxibustion, massage, cupping, foot bath and other therapies, are widely used in hypertension. Many studies at home and abroad have found that Tai Chi not only helps to reduce blood pressure, and improve headache and dizziness symptoms, but also can regulate vascular endothelial function, reduce the expression of inflammatory mediators, improve arteriosclerosis, reduce heart rate, reduce myocardial oxygen consumption, improve myocardial remodeling, and improve glucose and lipid metabolism. Chinese Health Qigong Association suggests popularizing Baduanjin in the community to improve blood pressure levels, clinical symptoms, and quality of life of patients with hypertension, which is beneficial to improving the activity tolerance of patients with heart disease. It is found that systolic blood pressure can be reduced by 13 mmHg and diastolic blood pressure by 6.13 mmHg after practicing Baduanjin for 3 months to 1 year.

As the most widely used non-medical therapy in TCM, acupuncture can not only improve the clinical symptoms of patients with hypertension, but also steadily reduce blood pressure and reduce complications and target organ damage. In the aspect of syndrome differentiation and acupoint selection, *Expert Consensus on Diagnosis and Treatment of Hypertension with Traditional Chinese Medicine* points out that commonly used antihypertensive acupoints include Tàichōng (LR3), Xíngjiān (LR2), Yǒngquán (KI1), Yánglíngquán (GB34), Sānyīnjiāo (SP6), Zúsānlǐ (ST36), Fēnglóng (ST40), Tàixī (KI3), and Qǔchí (LI11). Academician Shi Xuemin also found that acupuncture can effectively control blood pressure, take effect quickly and have a good duration of lowering blood pressure.

Massage can dredge meridians and harmonize qi and blood, and can also treat hypertension. Some studies have found that, based on conventional antihypertensive medicines, massage treatment for 20 days to 4 months can reduce systolic blood pressure by 6.92 mmHg and diastolic blood pressure by 3.63 mmHg. In addition, the clinical symptoms of vertigo, headache, soreness of the waist and knees, and dysphoria with feverish sensations in the chest can be significantly improved.

Foot bath is also one of the external treatments of TCM, which can activate qi and promote blood circulation, dredge meridians and increase blood circulation through thermal physical stimulation of warm water. Professor Deng Tietao, a great master of Chinese medicine, likes to use foot bath to treat hypertension, especially for hypertensive patients with exuberance of liver fire and hyperactivity of yang due to yin deficiency. Foot bath twice daily can not only improve blood pressure levels, but also improve dizziness. It is worth noting that in the foot bath process, we should keep warm and avoid the wind and cold. At the same time, people with skin diseases, burns and scalds are not suitable for foot bath.

References

ZHANG D Y, CHENG Y B, GUO Q H, et al. Treatment of masked hypertension with a Chinese herbal formula[J]. Circulation, 2020, 142: 1821-1830.

LAI X, DONG Z, WU S, et al. Efficacy and safety of Chinese herbal medicine compared with losartan for mild essential hypertension: a randomized, multicenter, double-blind, noninferiority trial Circulation: Cardiovascular Quality and Outcomes, 2022, 15 (3): e007923. doi: 10.1161/CIRCOUTCOMES. 121. 007923.

XIONG X J, WANG J. On TCM understanding of hypertension and prevention and treatment strategies of classic prescriptions[J]. Journal of Traditional Chinese Medicine, 2011, 52 (23): 1985-1989.

3 Arrhythmia

Many patients may have experienced palpitation, which is probably arrhythmia in medicine. Arrhythmia refers to any abnormality in the origin of heart impulse, heartbeat frequency and rhythm, and impulse conduction. In etiology, it can be caused by various organic cardiovascular diseases, medicine poisoning, electrolyte, and acid-base imbalance, and other factors. It can also appear in patients with vegetative nervous dysfunction without any underlying diseases.

According to the heart rate when an arrhythmia occurs, it can be divided into 2 categories: tachyarrhythmia and bradyarrhythmia. The former is seen in premature beating, tachycardia, atrial fibrillation, and ventricular fibrillation; the latter is common in sinus bradyarrhythmia and various conduction blocks.

In clinical diagnosis, it mainly depends on an electrocardiogram, but quite a few patients can make a preliminary diagnosis according to their medical history and signs. When the patient is having an attack, he/she should be asked in detail whether the heart rate is fast, whether the rhythm is chaotic, whether the heartbeat is regular, whether there is a sense of missing beat, whether there is hypotension, fainting, convulsion, angina pectoris, etc., which are helpful to judge the nature of arrhythmia.

In treatment, there are 2 types: medication and non-medication. Non-medication therapy includes radiofrequency catheter ablation for tachyarrhythmia, permanent pacemaker implantation for bradyarrhythmia, implantable cardioverter defibrillator for malignant ventricular arrhythmia, and so on. However, non-medication therapy requires high technical equipment, and the treatment cost is relatively expensive. Commonly used medicines for treating arrhythmia include sodium, potassium, calcium channel blockers, and beta-blockers. It is worth noting that these medicines often have a poor curative effect. Many medicines for "treating" arrhythmia have side effects, such as "causing" arrhythmia, damaging heart function, inducing heart failure, hypothyroidism, liver function damage, and even increased mortality. There is no Western medicine that can be used for a long time for slow arrhythmia. In recent years, the clinical value of TCM in treating arrhythmia has been gradually recognized by patients.

In TCM, arrhythmia belongs to the category of "palpitation". In etiology, the occurrence of this disease is mainly related to physical weakness, insufficiency of congenital endowment due to long-term illness, weak body, or malnutrition caused by long-term illness, excessive labor and sex life, diet and overstrain, addiction to eating fatty and greasy food, usual timidity due to deficiency of heart qi, sudden panic or emotional discomfort, excessive sorrow, attack by external pathogen, wind, cold and dampness pathogens, medicine poisoning, etc. In pathogenesis, arrhythmia is related to deficiency of blood, yin and yang, malnutrition of heart, or blockade of phlegm and fluid retention and static blood, and unsmooth heart vessel.

In modern clinical practice, classic prescriptions Zhigancao Decoction, Wendan Decoction, and Chinese patent medicine Shensong Yangxin Capsule are commonly used. Zhigancao Decoction comes from *Treatise on Cold Pathogenic Diseases*. In ancient times, this prescription was also called Fumai Decoction, which means it can make the disordered pulse rhythm return to normal. In the original text, Zhigancao Decoction is used to treat irregularly intermittent and regularly intermittent pulse and palpitation, and its primary effects are benefiting qi and nourishing yin, dredging yang and restoring pulse. Currently, this prescription has been widely used in clinic for patients with a series of arrhythmias, such as ventricular premature, atrial premature, and atrial fibrillation, which are characterized by an irregular heartbeat, palpitation, shortness of breath, red or mirror-like tongue, light color, and lack of fluid. In addition, we have found that this prescription can be used for some atrial fibrillation patients with transsinus and without thrombotic events.

Wendan Decoction recorded in *Treatise on Three Categories of Pathogenic Factors* in the Song Dynasty, is composed of Banxia (Pinelliae Rhizoma), Zhuru (Bambusae Caulis in Taenias), Zhishi (Aurantii Fructus Immaturus), Chenpi (Citri Reticulatae Rericarpium), Gancao (Glycyrrhizae Radix et Rhizoma), and Fuling (Poria). It has the effects of regulating qi-flow to eliminate phlegm, and harmonizing stomach and promoting bile flow. It is mainly used clinically to treat stagnated gallbladder qi with disturbing phlegm syndrome. People may be characterized by timidity, easiness to panic, palpitations, especially easiness to be frightened by the outside sound, but also accompanied by upset, egersis, night dreams, nightmares, nausea, headache, dizziness, epilepsy, white greasy tongue coating, stringy and slippery pulse. Many patients with arrhythmia will show the above symptoms. Wendan Ningxin Granule, an in-hospital preparation in Guang'anmen Hospital of China Academy of Chinese Medical Sciences, comes from Wendan Decoction, which is widely used in the clinic and is well received by patients.

Shensong Yangxin Capsule was developed by Academician Wu Yiling of the Chinese Academy of Engineering based on the philosophy of "qi-yin yang-five elements" of TCM. They put forward a new strategy of integrating regulation from "regulation" to "leveling". Shensong Yangxin Capsule are composed of Renshen (Ginseng Radix et Rhizoma), Maidong (Ophiopogonis Radix), Shanzhuyu (Corni Rructus), Danshen (Salviae Miltiorrhizae Radix et Rhizoma), Suanzaoren (Ziziphi Spinosae Semen), Sangjisheng (Taxilli Herba), Chishao (Paeoniae Radix Rubra), Tubiechong (Eupolyphaga Steleophaga), Gansong (Nardostachyos Radix et Rhizoma), Huanglian (Coptidis Rhizoma), Nanwuweizi (Schisandrae Sphenantherae Fructus), and Longgu (Os Draconis). It has the effects of benefiting qi and nourishing yin, promoting blood circulation for removing obstruction in collaterals, and clearing the heart for tranquillization. It can be used to treat premature ventricular beats of coronary heart disease. According to TCM syndrome differentiation, it belongs to the syndrome of deficiency of both qi and yin and stagnant blockade of heart blood collateral. Patients can show palpitation and uneasiness, shortness of breath, fatigue, aggravation after movement, chest oppression and pain, insomnia, dreaminess, night sweating, lethargy, and laziness to talk. Currently, Shensong Yangxin Capsule has completed the evidence-based study of multicenter, randomized, double-blind clinical trials of five diseases—premature ventricular beats, paroxysmal atrial fibrillation, bradyarrhythmia, mild and moderate cardiac insufficiency with premature ventricular beat, and sinus bradycardia with premature ventricular beat. Shensong Yangxin Capsule can regulate multi-ion and non-ion channels, regulate autonomic nerve, and improve sinus node function. In addition, it can also promote myocardial electrical conduction, improve myocardial blood supply and inhibit ventricular remodeling, protecting cardiac function. The medicine is taken orally, 2–4 capsules at a time, 3 times daily.

References

XIONG X J. Traceability of Zhigancao Decoction based on modern pathophysiology and CCU acute and critical cases and its clinical application of cardioversion, sinus conversion, hemostasis, platelet raising and deficiency tonifying [J]. China Journal of Chinese Materia Medica, 2019, 44 (18): 3842-3860.

4 Heart failure

Clinically, many patients with coronary heart disease and valvular heart disease have aggravated dyspnea and suffocation, edema of both lower limbs, and breathing difficulties after "catching a cold and suffering cold pathogen", and are diagnosed as "heart failure" after going to the hospital for examination. Heart failure refers to the dysfunction of systolic function or diastolic function of the heart, which can not thoroughly discharge the venous return blood volume from the heart, resulting in venous blood stasis and arterial blood perfusion deficiency, thus causing cardiac circulation disorder syndrome. Heart failure is not an independent disease, but the final stage of the development of heart disease. Most heart failure begins with left heart failure, manifested as pulmonary circulation congestion. The incidence of this disease is high, and the five-year survival rate is similar to that of a malignant tumor.

In etiology, almost all cardiovascular diseases will eventually lead to heart failure, including coronary atherosclerosis, hypertension, heart valve diseases, and so on. Based on heart disease, the sudden aggravation of heart failure mainly has inducing factors. Common inducements include: respiratory tract infection, rheumatic attack, tachyarrhythmia, such as atrial fibrillation and paroxysmal tachycardia, pregnancy, childbirth, excessively rapid infusion and excessive intake of sodium salt, resulting in increased cardiac load, digitalis poisoning, excessive physical activity and emotional excitement, and others, such as pulmonary embolism, anemia, papillary muscle insufficiency, etc. In autumn and winter, dyspnea and suffocation in many patients with chronic heart failure will worsen after suffering cold pathogen, complicated with a lung infection, and they will come to the hospital for treatment. Therefore, how to control infection and keep warm is particularly critical for patients with heart failure.

In clinical symptoms, breathing difficulties are the most common clinical symptom of left heart failure, manifested as exertional dyspnea, orthopnea, paroxysmal dyspnea at night, and so on. We can also see the decline in sports endurance and fatigue, etc. In the case of right heart failure, patients can also have abdominal or leg edema. Many patients came to see a doctor because they suddenly found edema in their lower limbs or decreased physical strength.

In clinical diagnosis, diagnosis can be made according to the previous medical history of primary cardiovascular diseases, such as coronary heart disease and hypertension, clinical symptoms of breathing difficulties, fatigue and edema of lower limbs during rest or exercise, and objective evidence, such as tachycardia, tachypnea, pulmonary rale, heart murmur, echocardiography and elevated NT-proBNP level, etc.

In clinical treatment, it has changed from short-term hemodynamic/pharmacological treatment schemes, such as diuresis, cardiotonic, and vasodilators, to long-term and restorative strategies based on neuroendocrine inhibitors. Although Western medicine has made significant progress in treatment, there are still some patients with recurrent heart failure, weak response to diuretics, and even diuretic resistance, and the improvement of dyspnea and suffocation, and edema is not ideal.

In TCM, heart failure belongs to the category of "edema" and "dyspnea syndrome". According to TCM, this situation is related to deficiency and decline of kidney yang, deficiency of primordial qi, blockade of heart blood, internal stagnation of fluid and internal blockade of static blood, which is the syndrome of deficient root cause and excessive manifestation and intermingled deficiency and excess. If it cannot be treated, the patient will suffer from repeated dyspnea and suffocation, and edema for a long time, which will easily lead to severe dyspnea depletion. This disease, which belongs to extreme yang qi deficiency, in essence, has already belonged to the ancient "consumptive disease". It is worth noting that in Western medicine, there are only treatment ideas and methods for diseases. However, there is a lack of tonifying deficiency for "deficiency syndrome". Deficiency syndrome and "tonifying deficiency" in TCM are effective supplements and perfections of diagnosis and treatment schemes for some Western medical diseases. We have found that cardiovascular diseases, such as refractory heart failure, dilated cardiomyopathy, ischemic cardiomyopathy, and valvular heart disease, belong to the traditional category of "consumptive disease". In this case, we recommend using semiliquid herbal extract to regulate chronic heart failure.

Semiliquid herbal extract, also known as tonifying ointment and decoction ointment, is a semi-fluid dosage form made by repeatedly decocting Chinese medicinal pieces, removing residue and extracting juice, evaporating, concentrating, adding auxiliary materials, and collecting ointment. Most ointments are designed for "deficiency syndrome" and "consumptive disease". Nowadays, most ointments are used in the clinic for "preventive treatment of disease", nourishment and aftercare, health maintenance and longevity, prevention of aging, and prolonging life to prevent and treat chronic diseases. In treating severe heart failure, dilated cardiomyopathy, ischemic cardiomyopathy, valvular heart disease, etc., taking supplementing ointment for a long time can not only effectively relieve symptoms and improve quality of life, but also improve heart structure and function, reduce diuretic dosage, reduce the frequency of hospitalization and achieve the purpose of secondary prevention. In the ointment, we often use Dangshen (Codonopsis Radix), Baizhu (Atractylodis Macrocephalae Rhizoma), Huangqi (Astragali Radix), and other Chinese medicinals, which can invigorate spleen and benefit qi to better improve the symptoms of fatigue and dyspnea and suffocation in patients with heart failure. We have treated a patient with valvular heart disease, tricuspid valvular deformity (Ebstein malformation), chronic heart failure, and cardiac function grade IV (NYHA grade). His NT-proBNP was 12,539 pg/ml, and heart failure occurred frequently. Moreover, he was hospitalized 6 times a year, with repeated attacks and repeated hospitalization. He was treated with ointment, which can warm yang and benefit qi, and was not hospitalized again for 2 years. The experience of treating heart failure with Chinese medicinals deserves attention.

References

XIONG X J, YOU H, SU K L. Secondary prevention of severe heart failure with Chinese medicinal tonifying ointment[J]. China Journal of Chinese Materia Medica, 2019, 44 (18): 3903-3907.

5 Viral myocarditis

Some children who are mistakenly thought of having a cold are often seen in the clinic, and they will not come to the hospital until they have severe chest oppression, palpitation, and other discomforts. They will have problems when doing electrocardiograms and taking blood to check myocardial enzymes, and are finally diagnosed with "viral myocarditis".

Viral myocarditis is a localized or diffuse acute or chronic inflammatory lesion of the myocardium caused by viral infection, which belongs to infectious myocardial disease. During the virus epidemic infection, about 5 % of patients will have myocarditis, and sporadic onset too. Among them, coxsackie virus group B virus is the dominant virus.

The clinical manifestations depend on the location and extent of myocardial lesions. Mild cases may not show any discomfort, while severe cases may show heart failure, cardiogenic shock and sudden death. 1–3 weeks before the onset of this disease, there is usually a history of upper respiratory tract or intestinal infection. Some patients will have a fever, soreness all over, sore throat, burnout and fatigue, nausea and vomiting, diarrhea, and other symptoms, and then have chest oppression, chest pain, dull pain in the precordial area, palpitation, dizziness, breathing difficulties, edema of lower limbs, and even Adams-Stokes syndrome; very few patients will show heart failure or cardiogenic shock.

In clinical diagnosis, the disease can be comsidered in combination with the history of prodromal infection, clinical manifestations, electrocardiogram, and myocardial injury markers, the diagnosis of this disease can be considered. However, the diagnosis of this disease depends on endocardial myocardial biopsy.

Although the disease can be clearly diagnosed, there is still a lack of specific treatment, and only myocardial nutrition and symptomatic treatment are the primary methods. Some patients will actively seek TCM treatment in the acute stage to speed up rehabilitation. Many patients come to see a doctor with chest oppression and palpitation after myocarditis. Taking Chinese medicinals can help relieve the clinical symptoms of chest oppression and palpitation.

In TCM, viral myocarditis belongs to the categories of "palpitation", "chest bi", "warm disease", etc., which are mainly related to exogenous warm-heat pathogenic toxin, entering from the outside to the inside and damaging the heart. The exogenous warm-heat pathogenic toxin is easy to consume qi and injure yin. Therefore, clinically, damage of both qi and yin of the heart is the root cause of viral myocarditis.

Classic prescriptions Zhigancao Decoction and Shengmai Powder are commonly used representative prescriptions for treating viral myocarditis. Zhigancao Decoction comes from the *Treatise on Cold Pathogenic Diseases*. The original text is mainly used for "irregularly intermittent and regularly intermittent pulse and palpitation". This suggests that in ancient times, it was a prescription for treating irregular pulse, palpitation, burnout, and fatigue, red and mirror-like tongue, little or no fur, or dry and thin tongue. Patients with viral myocarditis are prone to the above syndromes. Because this prescription has a remarkable effect on improving palpitation, it is often considered a special remedy for viral myocarditis. Mr. Yue Meizhong also likes to use this prescription to treat viral myocarditis.

Shengmai Powder is also a classic prescription of TCM, which is composed of Renshen (Ginseng Radix et Rhizoma), Maidong (Ophiopogonis Radix), and Wuweizi (Schisandrae Chinensis Fructus). This formula is a supplementing one and has the effects of benefiting qi for promoting production of fluid, and astringing yin and arresting sweating. Shengmai Powder can be used to treat the syndrome of damage of both qi and yin. Patients are characterized by profuse sweating and spirit fatigue, a tired body and fatigue, shortness of breath, laziness to talk, dry throat and thirst, dry red tongue with little fur, and feeble and rapid pulse. Some patients with viral myocarditis will show immobility and walking fatigue in the acute or recovery period, which is a typical indication of Shengmai Powder. Chinese patent medicine Shengmai Yin Oral Liquid comes from Shengmai Powder.

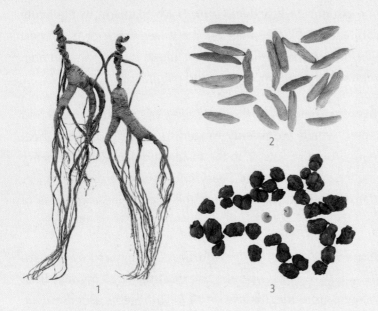

Shengmai Powder
1. Renshen; 2. Maidong;
3. Wuweizi.

In terms of prognosis, most patients can be cured after treatment, and only a few died of severe arrhythmia, acute heart failure, and cardiogenic shock in the acute stage. If rest is ignored or even treatment is delayed, some patients will develop into dilated cardiomyopathy. Clinically, we have seen young patients with a repeated sore throat, mistaken for a cold. It was not until they had chest oppression and palpitation, and dyspnea and suffocation for them to be unable to lie on their backs that they went to the doctor and were diagnosed with dilated cardiomyopathy, which was a pity.

6 Cardiomyopathy

Cardiomyopathy is an abnormal mechanical and electrical activity of the heart caused by different causes, manifested as ventricular hypertrophy or dilatation. Severe cardiomyopathy can lead to death or heart failure. Cardiomyopathy is usually divided into primary and secondary cardiomyopathy. Primary cardiomyopathy includes dilated cardiomyopathy, hypertrophic cardiomyopathy, restrictive cardiomyopathy, arrhythmogenic right ventricular cardiomyopathy, and unestablished cardiomyopathy. Secondary cardiomyopathy refers to cardiomyopathy as part of a systemic disease.

In etiology, the occurrence of cardiomyopathy is closely related to many factors. The pathogenesis of primary cardiomyopathy is unknown, while secondary cardiomyopathy is mainly related to infection, metabolic diseases, endocrine diseases, ischemia, allergy, and other factors.

In clinical symptoms, various cardiomyopathy symptoms are different. Dilated cardiomyopathy, which starts slowly, sometimes lasts for more than 10 years and is common among middle-aged people. Shortness of breath and edema are the main clinical symptoms in the clinic. Shortness of breath may occur initially after fatigue, and later during mild activity. Hypertrophic cardiomyopathy can occur without any discomfort, or it can also be manifested as palpitation, exertional dyspnea, precordial pain, easy fatigue, syncope, and even sudden death.

In clinical diagnosis, by combining medical history, physical examination, electrocardiogram, X-ray, echocardiography, coronary angiography, radionuclide ventriculography, and so on, diagnosis can be made.

The clinical treatment mainly includes etiological treatment and symptomatic treatment. It is worth noting that once cardiomyopathy develops, there will be changes in the systolic or diastolic function of the heart, most of which are difficult to reverse, especially when the ejection fraction is less than 30%. Although some patients may have no apparent clinical symptoms of chest oppression and suffocation, there is a high potential risk of sudden death. Most patients with cardiomyopathy actively seek TCM treatment to improve symptoms, improve quality of life, and reduce mortality.

According to TCM, cardiomyopathy belongs to the categories of "edema", "dyspnea syndrome", "chest bi", etc. In etiology, deficiency of heart qi or deficiency of heart-kidney yang is the internal cause; external pathogen invasion, overwork, disorder due to long-term disease, and so on are external causes.

Generally speaking, this disease is based on excessive manifestation and deficient root causes.

In clinical practice, Zhenwu Decoction, a famous classic prescription, is frequently used. Zhenwu Decoction comes from the *Treatise on Cold Pathogenic Diseases* in the Han Dynasty, which is composed of Fuling (Poria), Shaoyao (Paeoniae Radix Alba seu Rubra), Shengjiang (Zingiberis Rhizoma Recens), Fuzi (Aconiti Lateralis Radix Praeparata), and Baizhu (Atractylodis Macrocephalae Rhizoma). It has the effects of warming yang for diuresis. Zhenwu Decoction can be mainly used to treat syndrome of water overflowing due to yang deficiency. Patients with cardiomyopathy have dyspnea and suffocation and even can not lie on their backs, edema of both lower limbs, palpitation, dizziness, unstable standing, dysuria, less urine volume, light and fat tongue, teeth marks on the edge, white and slippery tongue fur, deep and thready pulse, etc., all of which belong to the indications of Zhenwu Decoction. We have found that the ejection fraction of some patients can be improved after taking Zhenwu Decoction for a long time. A patient with dilated cardiomyopathy was treated with an ejection fraction of 21%. Coronary angiography was performed to exclude coronary heart disease. During hospitalization, the patient was told that cardiac resynchronization therapy could be considered, but his family refused because of the high cost. After 2 years of treatment with Zhenwu Decoction, the ejection fraction increased to 48%. The reason why the patient's heart function could be improved is that he took Chinese medicinals over the years and could get rid of the heavy burden of cardiac resynchronization therapy.

References

XIONG X J. *Treatise on Cold Pathogenic Diseases* and acute and critical diseases—interpreting the connotation of classical provisions, the dosage of classical prescriptions, and the essence of six meridians based on severe cases of CCU and integration of Chinese and Western medicine[J]. China Journal of Chinese Materia Medica, 2018, 43 (12): 2413-2430.

Section 3

Digestive System Diseases

I Overview of digestive system diseases

People often say that "a good appetite is a blessing", but just "a good appetite" is not enough. The food eaten must be digested and absorbed smoothly, and finally, the garbage and waste can be discharged through feces, which is perfect. All this depends on whether our digestive system functions normally. Once any link of this "production line" breaks down, we suffer from so-called digestive system diseases.

In Western medicine, digestive system diseases are a group of systemic diseases, such as gastritis, peptic ulcer, gastric cancer, gastroesophageal reflux disease, esophageal cancer, ulcerative colitis, and so on. In addition to nausea, vomiting, acid regurgitation, abdominal pain, diarrhea, hematochezia, and other digestive system symptoms, clinical manifestations are often accompanied by other systemic or systemic symptoms. In clinical diagnosis, besides the chief complaint, it is necessary to combine laboratory examination, endoscopy, abdominal B-ultrasound, plain abdominal radiography, abdominal and pelvic CT or MR, and pathological biopsy results before the diagnosis can be made.

In clinical treatment, commonly used treatment methods include medical therapy, endoscopic therapy, surgical treatment, radiotherapy and chemotherapy, and targeted immune therapy. However, it is found that there are still some patients whose symptoms are not improved sufficiently, and there are still apparent discomforts, such as anorexia, nausea, poor appetite, and diarrhea, so they seek TCM treatment. TCM has apparent advantages in improving symptoms related to digestive system diseases, regulating the constitution and improving the quality of life.

According to symptoms, digestive system diseases belong to the categories of "stomachache", "abdominal pain", "dysphagia", "diarrhea", "constipation", etc., and these diseases are located in the spleen, stomach, and intestine. This section will focus on TCM understanding and treatment of functional dyspepsia, gastroesophageal reflux disease, gastritis, constipation, ulcerative colitis, and chronic diarrhea.

‖ Treatises on digestive system diseases

1 Functional dyspepsia

Functional dyspepsia is the most common functional gastrointestinal disease in the clinic, which is caused by the dysfunction of stomach and duodenum. Patients often complain of "a little food feeding them up", "a normal amount of food making them full and uncomfortable after a meal", nausea, loss of appetite, hiccup, and "burning pain" in the middle and upper abdomen. But no organic lesions were found when they went to the hospital for examination.

In clinical diagnosis, it is necessary to make sure that the patient has no symptoms and signs suggesting organic diseases, such as emaciation, anemia, hematemesis, melena, abdominal mass, and jaundice, exclude organic diseases of the digestive tract, and finally make a precise diagnosis in combination with specific indigestion symptoms, blood biochemistry, gastrointestinal endoscopy, and other examination results.

In clinical treatment, symptomatic medical treatment and adjustment of living and eating habits are the primary methods. However, there are still some patients whose symptoms still recur after taking medicines and changing their living habits, which leads to insomnia, anxiety, depression, and other psychological problems.

TCM has certain clinical advantages in treating functional dyspepsia. In TCM, functional dyspepsia belongs to the categories of "stomachache", "distention and fullness" and "hiccup". In etiology, it is mainly induced by being attacked by external pathogen, improper diet, and poor emotions; in pathogenesis, it is mainly related to dysfunction of spleen and stomach in ingestion and transportation and imbalance of ascending and descending.

In clinical treatment, Simo Decoction Oral Liquid and acupuncture therapy are commonly used. Simo Decoction comes from Yan Yonghe's *Re-ordering Yan's Jisheng Prescription* in the Song Dynasty. It is composed of 4 Chinese medicinals: Tiantai Wuyao (Linderae Radix), Chenxiang (Aquilariae Lignum Resinatum), Renshen (Ginseng Radix et Rhizoma), and Binglang (Arecae Semen). It has the effects of promoting circulation of qi for lowering adverse qi, and removing food retention and relieving pain. This prescription can treat the distension and fullness of abdomen, pain, poor defecation, and other symptoms caused by food retention and qi stagnation. It can also treat postoperative abdominal distension in adults. Functional dyspepsia patients with symptoms of anorexia, poor appetite, distension and fullness in the epigastrium and abdomen, abdominal pain, and constipation can take this prescription. Now, Simo Decoction Oral Liquid has been developed from this prescription. The administration and dosage is to take 20 ml orally, 3 times daily for 1 week. A systematic review of 27 clinical studies involving 2,713 patients with dyspepsia, showed that Simotang Oral Liquid can not only shorten the time of gastric emptying, improve the rate of gastric emptying, but also reduce the recurrence rate of functional dyspepsia.

In addition to the above medical therapy, acupuncture therapy is commonly used to relieve the symptoms of functional dyspepsia. Common clinical acupoints include Shàngwǎn (CV13), Zhōngwǎn (CV12), Xiàwǎn (CV10), Nèiguān (PC6), Dànzhōng (CV17), Tiānshū (ST25), Zúsānlǐ (ST36), Liángqiū (ST34), etc. On this basis, acupoint selection of TCM syndrome types is carried out. A randomized, controlled, and clinical study involving 278 patients with functional dyspepsia showed that compared with the sham acupuncture group, acupuncture treatment 3 times a week for 4 weeks could effectively relieve the 3 primary symptoms of fullness after meals, early satiety, and epigastric distension, and no recurrence was found after 12 weeks of follow-up after treatment.

References

HU Y, BAI Y, HUA Z, et al. Effect of Chinese patent medicine Si-Mo-Tang oral liquid for functional dyspepsia: a systematic review and meta-analysis of randomized controlled trials[J]. PLoS One, 2017, 12 (2): e0171878.

YANG J W, WANG L Q, ZOU X, et al. Effect of acupuncture for postprandial distress syndrome: a randomized clinical trial[J]. Ann Intern Med, 2020, 172 (12): 777-785.

2 Gastroesophageal reflux disease

We often see such people around us who sit restless after a meal, repeatedly complaining of "a burning pain in the stomach", "heartburn" and "daring not to belch, hiccup reversing sour water", "the sour water burning their throat, and wanting to cough", while others are comfortably sitting or lying. If relatives and friends around us have the above discomfort symptoms, they must be alert to a disease—gastroesophageal reflux disease (GERD).

GERD is a disease in which the contents of the stomach and duodenum flow back into the esophagus, causing discomfort or complications. Under normal circumstances, the contents of the gastroduodenum will not flow back into the esophagus. Long-term smoking, drinking, overeating, excessive eating of high-sugar, high-fat, spicy, and stimulating food, or taking some stimulant medicines for a long time lead to prolonged transient relaxation of the esophagus, abnormal esophageal peristalsis, and destruction of esophageal mucosal defense barrier. The contents of the gastroduodenum will "go upstream" to the esophagus. Because reflux contains strong acidic components such as gastric acid and pepsin, it will cause esophageal mucosa damage to varying degrees, and even mucosal erosion and ulcer.

In clinical symptoms, reflux and heartburn are the most common and most typical. They usually appear about 1 hour after a meal, and can be aggravated by lying on one's back, bending over, and sleeping at night. Some patients also have acid regurgitation and chest pain. Some patients also showed pharyngeal foreign body sensation, blockage sensation, irritant dry cough or asthma, and even took this as the first symptom. No abnormality was found in the respiratory specialist examination, and finally, they were diagnosed GERD.

In clinical diagnosis, proton pump inhibitors (such as omeprazole) can be given as experimental treatment. Moreover, if the symptoms are relieved, it can be preliminarily diagnosed as this disease. Of course, it is necessary to combine the results of gastroscopy, esophagography, and 24-hour esophageal pH monitoring, and exclude other diseases of the digestive system and other systemic diseases causing related symptoms before the diagnosis can be made.

Clinically, the treatment includes lifestyle adjustment, medical treatment (acid inhibitor, gastrointestinal motility promoting medicine, antacid), surgery, and so on. However, although some patients have been treated with Western medicine orally for a long time, the symptoms of acid regurgitation and heartburn persist. Thus, they turn to TCM for treatment. TCM has certain clinical advantages in relieving symptoms related to GERD, reducing recurrence frequency, and improving quality of life.

In TCM, this disease belongs to the category of "acid regurgitation". In etiology, it is mainly related to eating disorders and irregular work and rest. In pathogenesis, it is related to liver qi invading stomach, and failure of stomach qi to descend.

In clinical treatment, classic prescriptions such as Xiaochaihu Decoction and Wuzhuyu Decoction are commonly used. Xiaochaihu Decoction comes from *Treatise on Cold Pathogenic Diseases* written by Zhang Zhongjing, a medical sage. It is composed of 7 Chinese medicinals, including Chaihu (Bupleuri Radix), Huangqin (Scutellariae Radix), Banxia (Pinelliae Rhizoma), Shengjiang (Zingiberis Rhizoma Recens), Renshen (Ginseng Radix et Rhizoma), Dazao (Jujubae Fructus) and Gancao (Glycyrrhizae Radix et Rhizoma). It has the effect of reconciling Shaoyang. Gastroesophageal reflux is accompanied by dry mouth and a bitter taste, burning sensation behind the sternum, pharyngeal discomfort, chronic cough, or by loss of appetite, dysphoria, nausea, etc. Xiaochaihu Decoction can be selected. According to the clinical research of *World Journal of Gastroenterololy*, Xiaochaihu Decoction can not only improve the contractility of the lower esophageal sphincter and reduce ineffective swallowing in patients with mild to moderate GERD, but also significantly reduce the recurrence rate within 3 months. Moreover, its effect is similar to proton pump inhibitors.

Wuzhuyu Decoction is also from the *Treatise on Cold Pathogenic Diseases* written by Zhang Zhongjing. It is composed of 4 Chinese medicinals: Wuzhuyu (Euodiae Fructus), Shengjiang (Zingiberis Rhizoma Recens), Renshen (Ginseng Radix et Rhizoma), and Dazao (Jujubae Fructus). It has the effects of warming the spleen and stomach and supplementing deficiency, and lowering adverse qi and arresting vomiting. This prescription is suitable for patients with nausea and the desire to vomit, or retching, or vomiting acid water, or vomiting cold and thin water after eating, accompanied by chest oppression, stomach discomfort, pain in the top of the head, fear of cold, cold limbs, diarrhea, irritability, and other symptoms. A randomized, controlled and clinical trial involving 90 patients with GERD showed that compared with using omeprazole alone, adding Wuzhuyu Decoction not only improved reflux and heartburn symptoms, but also lasted longer.

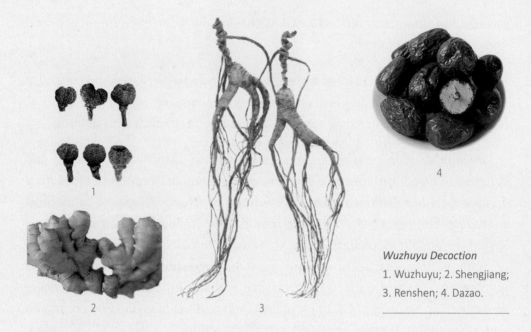

Wuzhuyu Decoction
1. Wuzhuyu; 2. Shengjiang;
3. Renshen; 4. Dazao.

References

XU L Y, YU B Y, CEN L S. New treatment for gastroesophageal reflux disease: Traditional Chinese medicine Xiaochaihu decoction[J]. World J Gastroenterol, 2022, 28 (11): 1184-1186.

SHIH Y S, TSAI C H, LI T C, et al. Effect of wu zhu yu tang on gastroesophageal reflux disease: randomized, double-blind, placebo-controlled trial[J]. Phytomedicine, 2019, 56: 118-125.

3 Chronic gastritis

Chronic gastritis refers to chronic inflammatory lesions of gastric mucosa caused by various factors. The most common cause is *Helicobacter pylori* infection. In addition, some medicines, alcohol, autoimmunity, aging, etc. can also induce it. Most adults have slight superficial inflammation of gastric mucosa, but most have no apparent discomfort.

In clinical symptoms, chronic gastritis is often manifested as indigestion symptoms, such as middle and upper abdominal discomfort, fullness, dull pain, slow pain, burning sensation, loss of appetite, nausea, pantothenic acid, belching, etc., but it lacks specificity. Severe cases may present with general weakness, anorexia, anemia, weight loss, hematemesis, melena, etc., and even progress to gastric cancer.

In clinical diagnosis, gastroscopy and histological examination are the key to diagnosis, and clinical manifestations alone cannot make a specific diagnosis.

In clinical treatment, medicine intervention is the primary method. For *Helicobacter pylori*-positive patients, "quadruple therapy" is routinely used. In addition, it also includes symptomatic treatment, correction of living and eating habits, etc. After the above intervention measures, the symptoms of most patients can be significantly relieved. However, some patients still have antibiotic intolerance, *Helicobacter pylori* is positive again after medicine withdrawal, and symptoms are not relieved during treatment. Thus, they turn to TCM for help. TCM has a certain curative effect on improving the clinical symptoms of chronic gastritis.

In TCM, chronic gastritis belongs to the categories of "stomachache", "distention and fullness" and "vomiting". In etiology, it is related to being attacked by external pathogen, improper diet, emotional disorder, and so on. In pathogenesis, it is mainly related to the dysfunction of spleen and stomach, imbalance of ascending and descending, the obstruction of stomach qi, or adverse rising of stomach qi.

In clinical treatment, Xiaochaihu Decoction and Berberine Tablet are commonly used. Xiaochaihu Decoction comes from *Treatise on Cold Pathogenic Diseases* written by Zhang Zhongjing, a medical sage. It is composed of 7 Chinese medicinals, including Chaihu (Bupleuri Radix), Huangqin (Scutellariae Radix), Banxia (Pinelliae Rhizoma), Shengjiang (Zingiberis Rhizoma Recens), Renshen (Ginseng Radix et Rhizoma), Dazao (Jujubae Fructus) and Gancao (Glycyrrhizae Radix et Rhizoma). It has the effect of reconciling Shaoyang. This prescription is suitable for patients with chronic gastritis, such as loss of appetite, nausea, belching, fullness in the middle and upper abdomen, or accompanied by dry mouth, a bitter taste, and dysphoria. Experimental studies have proved that Xiaochaihu Decoction can not only effectively inhibit *Helicobacter pylori*, but also show preventive and protective effects on stomach injury caused by alcohol.

Berberine Tablet is one of the most well-known medicines for treating diarrhea, which is favored by the public because of their low price, and convenience to take and carry. Berberine, also known as berberine hydrochloride, is a quaternary ammonium alkaloid isolated from Chinese medicinal—Huanglian (Coptidis Rhizoma), the main antibacterial component of Huanglian (Coptidis Rhizoma). Besides treating diarrhea, Berberine Tablet is also commonly used in treating chronic gastritis. Berberine is suitable for patients with chronic gastritis accompanied by diarrhea, thirst, red eyes, toothache, dysphoria and insomnia. The dosage for adults is 1–3 tablets each time, 3 times daily. Clinical studies have proved that berberine can effectively treat chronic atrophic gastritis caused by *Helicobacter pylori*.

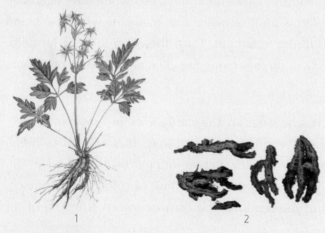

Huanglian
1. Source plant;
2. decoction pieces.

References

CHEN X, HU L J, WU H H, et al. Anti-*Helicobacter pylori* and anti-inflammatory effects and constituent analysis of modified Xiaochaihutang for the treatment of chronic gastritis and gastric ulcer[J]. Evid Based Complement Alternat Med, 2018, 2018: e6810369.

YANG T, WANG R L, LIU H H, et al. Berberine regulates macrophage polarization through IL-4-STAT6 signaling pathway in *Helicobacter pylori*-induced chronic atrophic gastritis[J]. Life Sci, 2021, 266: e118903.

4 Constipation

With the development of society, more and more people around us are distressed by constipation. The so-called constipation refers to the reduction of defecation frequency (less than 3 times a week), dry and hard feces and difficulty in defecation (laborious defecation, difficult excretion, incomplete defecation, time-consuming defecation, and manual assistance needed in defecation). When constipation lasts more than 12 weeks, it is called chronic constipation. Constipation is not only a defecation problem, but also causes psychological problems such as anxiety, irritability, and insomnia, which seriously affect the quality of life and work efficiency.

In etiology, the most common inducement includes terrible living habits and social psychological factors. The former includes eating too little, refined food, high calories, insufficient intake of fruits and vegetables, being sedentary, terrible defecation habits, and so on. Social psychological factors mainly refer to autonomic nervous dysfunction, intestinal peristalsis disorder, or broken defecation rules caused by interpersonal relationships, work pressure and emergencies. In addition, complications of some diseases (such as cerebral infarction, depression, diabetes, hypothyroidism), adverse reactions to some medicines, and surgery may cause constipation.

In terms of clinical symptoms, in addition to a series of manifestations mentioned above, there are also other symptoms including common lower abdominal pain, loss of appetite, fatigue, dizziness, dysphoria, insomnia, etc. Some patients may have anal pain, anal fissure, hemorrhoids, and anal inflammation due to forced defecation. Patients can voluntarily touched the cord, which is a long time stored stool in the lower left abdomen.

In clinical diagnosis, in addition to medical history, clinical symptoms and lifestyle, etc., it is necessary to combine plain abdominal film, gastrointestinal endoscopy, colon transit test, and other examination methods to clarify the etiology and final diagnosis of constipation. If the relevant auxiliary examination does not indicate organic lesions, it is diagnosed as functional constipation. Patients with hematochezia, occult blood positive stool, fever, anemia, vomiting, emaciation, and other symptoms should be thoroughly examined.

In clinical treatment, besides guiding patients to develop good living and defecation habits, medical therapy is a common means, including laxatives, medicines for promoting gastrointestinal motility, and medicines for regulating intestinal flora. We have found that there is apparent effect at the initial stage of medication in some patients. Over time, the effect gradually deteriorates or even becomes ineffective, resulting in secondary constipation. Or defecation is normal when taking medication; once the medication is stopped, constipation recurs, which brings significant pain and psychological burden to patients. Some patients will turn to TCM for treatment.

In TCM, the symptoms of "constipation" disease are consistent with constipation referred to in Western medicine. In etiology, it is mainly related to being attacked by external pathogen, eating disorders, poor emotions, and physical weakness after illness. In pathogenesis, most belong to pathogen stagnation in the large intestine, obstruction of fu-viscera qi, or impaired warmth and moistening of the intestine and pushing weakness, leading to abnormal conduction function of the large intestine.

In clinical treatment, the classic prescription Maziren Pill and acupuncture therapy are commonly used. Maziren Pill comes from *Treatise on Cold Pathogenic Diseases* written by Zhang Zhongjing, a medical sage. It consists of 7 Chinese medicinals: Houpo (Magnoliae Officinalis Cortex), Zhishi (Aurantii Fructus Immaturus), Maziren (Cannabis Fructus), Baishao (Paeoniae Radix Alba), Dahuang (Rhei Radix et Rhizoma), Xingren (Armeniacae Semen Amarum) and Baimi (Mel). Maziren Pill has the effects of moistening the intestine and purging heat, and activating qi and relaxing bowels. The medicine can treat constipation of gastrointestinal dryness-heat type, characterized by dry stool, abdominal distension, abdominal pain, dry mouth and halitosis, little yellow and burning urine, or accompanied by a red face, hot body, dysphoria, vexation, red tongue and yellow fur. Clinical studies have proved that Maziren Pill can effectively relieve functional constipation. Its mechanism is related to down-regulating oleamide levels, promoting intestinal peristalsis.

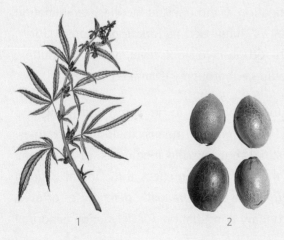

Huomaren
1. Source plant;
2. decoction pieces.

Clinically, besides taking medicine, acupuncture has a noticeable curative effect in treating constipation. A clinical study on patients with functional constipation led by Liu Zhishun, director of the acupuncture department of Guang'anmen Hospital, showed that, compared with the sham acupuncture group, electroacupuncture was performed at bilateral Tiānshū (ST25), Fùjié (SP14) and Shàngjùxū (ST37) for 30 minutes each time, and the course of treatment was 8 weeks. During the treatment, the constipation symptoms of patients were relieved, the number of spontaneous defecation increased, and the quality of life improved. There was no repetition in the follow-up. Its mechanism may be related to the activation of the parasympathetic nerve and the enhancement of colon peristalsis. The above research was published in the *Annals of Internal Medicine*, an authoritative international medical journal, and attracted international medical attention.

References

HUANG T, ZHAO L, LIN C Y,et al. Chinese herbal medicine (MaZiRenWan) improves bowel movement in functional constipation through down-regulating oleamide[J]. Front Pharmacol, 2020,10: 1570.

LIU Z S, YAN S Y, WU J N, et al. Acupuncture for chronic severe functional constipation: a randomized trial[J]. Ann Intern Med, 2016,165 (11): 761-769.

5 Ulcerative colitis

Ulcerative colitis is a chronic nonspecific intestinal inflammatory disease, and its etiology has not been clarified. Currently, it is considered that this disease is related to intestinal immune imbalance, intestinal mucosal barrier destruction, and intestinal mucosal persistent inflammatory injury caused by environmental factors, genetic factors, and intestinal microecological changes.

On the lesion site, the disease mainly starts from the rectum, with retrograde upward involvement of the colon and even the terminal ileum. The lesions are distributed continuously and diffusely, mainly damaging the mucosa and submucosa of the large intestine. In severe cases, the whole intestinal wall may be involved, complicated with intestinal perforation, toxic megacolon, abdominal abscess, and so on.

In clinical manifestations, the typical symptoms of this disease include recurrent diarrhea, mucous pus and bloody stool, and abdominal pain, which generally alternate between the attacking period and the remission period. Some patients may be accompanied by tenesmus, abdominal distension, loss of appetite, nausea and vomiting, fever, emaciation, anemia, and other malnutrition symptoms. Parenteral manifestations such as peripheral arthritis, recurrent oral ulcer and erythema nodularis can also be seen.

In clinical diagnosis, colonoscopy is the key to the diagnosis and differential diagnosis of this disease. If necessary, mucosal biopsy should be performed. If accompanied by fever, mucous pus, and bloody stool, blood routine, erythrocyte sedimentation rate, and fecal pathogen examination are needed to further clarify the stage of the disease and judge whether it is complicated with infection.

In clinical treatment, anti-inflammatory, immunosuppressive and symptomatic treatment are the primary methods, and acute and severe patients can undergo surgical treatment when necessary. Generally, mild patients have a good prognosis, but for elderly patients and patients with frequent attacks, hormone ineffectiveness, hormone dependence, gastrointestinal complications, bone marrow suppression, and other disadvantages often lead to repeated attacks. TCM treatment of ulcerative colitis has certain advantages in improving clinical symptoms and reducing attack frequency.

In TCM, ulcerative colitis belongs to the category of "dysentery". In etiology, it is related to exogenous seasonal pathogen and an unclean diet. In pathogenesis, most are caused by pathogen accumulating in intestines, the coagulation and stagnation of qi and blood, damage of blood collaterals of the large intestine lipid membrane, and conduction disorder.

In clinical treatment, the classic prescriptions Shaoyao Decoction and Chinese patent medicine Berberine Tablet are commonly used. Shaoyao Decoction comes from *Collection of Writings on the Mechanism of Disease, Suitability of Qi, and the Safeguarding of Life as Discussed in the 'Basic Questions'*, which is composed of 9 Chinese medicinals: Baishao (Paeoniae Radix Alba), Binglang (Arecae Semen), Dahuang (Rhei Radix et Rhizoma), Huangqin (Scutellariae Radix), Huanglian (Coptidis Rhizoma), Danggui (Angelicae Sinensis Radix), Rougui (Cinnamomi Cortex), Gancao (Glycyrrhizae Radix et Rhizoma) and Muxiang (Aucklandiae Radix). It has the effects of clearing zang-fu viscera heat, clearing heat and eliminating dampness, and regulating qi and harmonizing blood. It is mainly used for damp-heat dysentery. Moreover, it is suitable for ulcerative colitis, manifested as abdominal pain, mucous pus and bloody stool with red and white dischages, accompanied by tenesmus, burning and hot anus, little yellow urine with burning and hot sensation, and yellow and greasy tongue fur, etc. Experimental studies have confirmed that Shaoyao Decoction has a protective effect on ulcerative colitis and can maintain the integrity of the intestinal mucosal barrier. Its mechanism may be related to inhibiting MKP1/NF-κ B/NLRP3 pathway.

Berberine Tablet is a well-known Chinese patent medicine for treating diarrhea. Berberine, also known as berberine hydrochloride, is the primary antibacterial component of Huanglian. Berberine is suitable for ulcerative colitis patients with recurrent diarrhea, smelly stool, mucus pus and blood, abdominal pain, tenesmus, burning and hot anus, dry mouth, a bitter taste, dysphoria, and insomnia, or discomfort in the middle and upper abdomen, vomiting, acid regurgitation, and hiccup. The dosage of berberine is 1–3 tablets for adults, 3 times daily. Experimental studies have confirmed that berberine can activate the IL-25-ILC2-IL-13 immune pathway, promote the differentiation of intestinal stem cells and repair the intestinal mucosal barrier damage in ulcerative colitis.

References

WEI Y Y, FAN Y M, GA Y, et al. Shaoyao decoction attenuates DSS-induced ulcerative colitis, macrophage and NLRP3 inflammasome activation through the MKP1/NF-κB pathway[J]. Phytomedicine, 2021, 92: e153743.

XIONG X, CHENG Z, WU F, et al. Berberine in the treatment of ulcerative colitis: a possible pathway through Tuft cells[J]. Biomed Pharmacother, 2021, 134: e111129.

6 Chronic diarrhea

Chronic diarrhea refers to increased frequency of defecation (>3 times/day), or the increased volume of stool (>200g/day), or thin stool (water content >85%), and the disease course of more than 4 weeks, or long-term recurrent attacks. People often say that they often "have trouble with their stomach" and "have tough enteritis". In fact, not all chronic diarrhea is related to enteritis. From the etiological point of view, the gastrointestinal tract, liver and gallbladder, pancreas, and many other diseases can cause chronic diarrhea, which is why some patients have not seen improvement according to enteritis treatment for many years.

In pathogenesis and clinical symptoms, chronic diarrhea can be divided into the following 4 types: osmotic diarrhea, secretory diarrhea, exudative diarrhea, and dyskinetic diarrhea. Osmotic diarrhea is caused by eating indigestible food, food intolerance or taking certain medicines, which leads to a large amount of body fluid water entering the intestinal cavity. Generally, diarrhea is relieved or stopped after fasting. Secretory diarrhea is caused by enhanced secretion function of the intestinal mucosa, weakened absorption, and increased net secretion of water and electrolyte in the intestinal cavity. It is characterized by increased stool volume, and watery stool, no pus and blood, which can't be relieved by fasting. Exudative diarrhea, also known as inflammatory diarrhea, is caused by inflammation, necrosis, and exudation of intestinal mucosa caused by infectious (bacteria, viruses, parasites, etc.) or non-infectious (autoimmune diseases, tumors, etc.) factors, characterized by exudation or blood components in feces, and even gross pus and blood. Dyskinetic diarrhea is caused by excessive intestinal peristalsis and insufficient water absorption and electrolytes. Its characteristics include acute stool, unformed stool, accompanied by abdominal pain, and bowel sounds. Common inducements include suffering cold pathogen, diabetic complications, gastrointestinal motility medicines, hyperthyroidism, and other metabolic diseases.

In clinical diagnosis, the most critical thing is to clarify the etiology of chronic diarrhea. It is necessary to combine the medical history, clinical manifestations, abdominal B-ultrasound, gastrointestinal endoscopy, stool routine + occult blood, blood biochemistry, tumor markers, and other examination results, to clarify the etiology, lesion site, and final diagnosis.

Clinical treatment mainly relies on drug therapy, including causative treatment and symptomatic treatment. Commonly used medicines include antibiotics, probiotics, antidiarrheal medicines, intestinal peristalsis inhibitors, and so on. However, some patients still have no noticeable symptom relief, so they turn to TCM treatment. TCM has a certain curative effect in improving chronic diarrhea symptoms and quality of life.

In TCM, chronic diarrhea belongs to the category of "diarrhea". In etiology, it is mainly related to being attacked by external pathogen, eating disorders, emotion and internal damage, and overstrain and physical weakness. In pathogenesis, most cases are exuberance of dampness due to spleen deficiency and spleen and stomach failing in transportation and transformation.

In clinical treatment, the classic prescriptions Shenling Baizhu Powder and Fuzi Lizhong Pill are commonly used. Shenling Baizhu Powder comes from *Prescriptions of the Bureau of Taiping People's Welfare Pharmacy* in the Song Dynasty. It is composed of 10 Chinese medicinals, including Baibiandou (Lablab Semen Album), Baizhu (Atractylodis Macrocephalae Rhizoma), Fuling (Poria), Gancao (Glycyrrhizae Radix et Rhizoma), Jiegeng (Platycodonis Radix), Lianzi (Nelumbinis Semen), Renshen (Ginseng Radix et Rhizoma), Sharen (Amomi Fructus), Shanyao (Dioscoreae Rhizoma) and Yiyiren (Coicis Semen). It has the effects of invigorating spleen and stomach, and benefiting lung qi. It is suitable for chronic diarrhea with repeated attacks, thin feces, abdominal distension, active bowel sounds, loss of appetite, shortness of breath, cough, chest oppression, fatigued limbs, and emaciation. This prescription has been made into the Chinese patent medicine preparation—Shenling Baizhu Granule. The dosage and administration is usually 1 bag (3 g) each time, 3 times daily. Experimental studies have shown that Shenling Baizhu Powder can alleviate lactose-induced diarrhea, and its mechanism may be related to regulating intestinal absorption function and intestinal mucosal ultrastructure.

Fuzi Lizhong Pill, also from *Prescriptions of the Bureau of Taiping People's Welfare Pharmacy* in the Song Dynasty, is composed of 5 Chinese medicinals: Fuzi (Aconiti Lateralis Radix Praeparata), Renshen (Ginseng Radix et Rhizoma), Ganjiang (Zingiberis Rhizoma), Gancao (Glycyrrhizae Radix et Rhizoma) and Baizhu (Atractylodis Macrocephalae Rhizoma). It has the effects of warming the spleen and stomach and invigorating the spleen. It is mainly used for treating the syndrome of deficient cold of the spleen and stomach. It is suitable for patients with chronic diarrhea, accompanied by repeated attacks of diarrhea, thin feces, no terrible smell or slight fishy smell, no tenesmus, burning and hot anus, cold abdominal pain, abdominal distension, hyperactive bowel sounds, poor diet, a taste for hot food, cold hands, and feet, or vomiting, hiccup and acid regurgitation, etc. The routine dosage and administration method is 1 pill at a time, 2–3 times daily. Experimental studies have shown that the mechanism of Fuzi Lizhong Pill in treating diarrhea may be related to regulating the diversity and community structure of intestinal flora and regulating inflammation and the immune system.

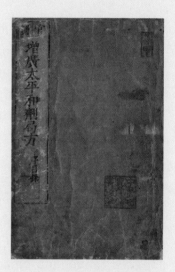

Beneficial Formulas from the Taiping Imperial Pharmacy
(Zēng Guǎng Tài Píng Huì Mín Hé Jì Jú Fāng, 增广太平惠民和剂局方)
Preserved in China Academy of Chinese Medical Sciences (CACMS)

References

JI H J, KANG N, CHEN T, et al. Shen-ling-bai-zhu-san, a spleen-tonifying Chinese herbal formula, alleviates lactose-induced chronic diarrhea in rats[J]. J Ethnopharmacol, 2019, 231: 355-362.

ZHEN Z, XIA L, YOU H, et al. An integrated gut microbiota and network pharmacology study on Fuzi-Lizhong Pill for treating diarrhea-predominant irritable bowel syndrome[J]. Front Pharmacol, 2021, 12: e746923.

Section 4
Urinary System Diseases

| Overview of urinary system diseases

Some people suddenly find their eyelids swollen and shiny when they get up in the morning. If they have some health awareness, they may think of performing a urine routine and checking whether they have kidney disease. We have seen a competent graduate student who suddenly developed facial edema, which was later diagnosed as acute glomerulonephritis.

The urinary system mainly comprises kidney, ureter, bladder, urethral canal, and related blood vessels and nerves. Clinical common urinary system diseases include glomerulonephritis, IgA nephropathy, chronic renal failure, urinary tract infection, urinary incontinence, and other diseases. Its clinical manifestations are diverse. Renal diseases can be manifested as hematuria, proteinuria, edema, hypertension, renal function damage, etc. Urinary tract infection can be manifested as frequent micturition, urgent micturition, painful micturition, fever, low back pain, and abnormal changes in urine properties.

In treatment, commonly used medicines include antibiotics, diuretics, hormones, cytotoxic medicines, and so on. However, most urinary system diseases are complicated, lingering, and challenging to heal, and the clinical effect is unsatisfactory. We have found that patients often feel anxious due to significant diseases such as chronic renal failure. Even if urine protein, occult urine blood, and mild creatinine increase are found in physical examination, patients will be nervous and seek medical advice everywhere. Many patients will choose TCM treatment.

Urinary system diseases belong to the "kidney system" syndrome of TCM, pertaining to the categories of "edema", "strangury", "turbid urine" and "anuria and vomiting". TCM believes that this kind of disease is located in the kidney and bladder, and its etiology and pathogenesis are closely related to deficiency of spleen and kidney, dysfunction of qi transformation, dampness-heat amassment, and water and liquid failing in transportation and transformation, etc. In TCM treatment, the primary treatment principle is to tonify and benefit spleen and kidney or clear heat and promote diuresis. At the same time, treatment based on syndrome differentiation should be practiced according to specific conditions. In each treatise, we will introduce the characteristics and advantages of TCM treatment around acute glomerulonephritis, IgA nephropathy, chronic renal failure, urinary tract infection, and urinary incontinence.

‖ Treatises on urinary system diseases

1 Acute glomerulonephritis

Clinically, we often see some patients, after suffering from tonsillitis, scarlet fever or impetigo, suddenly presented with facial or lower limb edema, possibly accompanied by proteinuria, gross hematuria, and hypertension. This may be secondary to acute glomerulonephritis after infection.

Acute glomerulonephritis, referred to as acute nephritis, can occur at any age, especially in children and adolescents aged 5–15. It is more common after acute streptococcal infection, and often starts acutely 2 weeks after infection. In recent years, due to the widespread use of antibiotics, and other reasons, studies have shown that the incidence of antibiotics has shown a downward trend.

In terms of clinical symptoms, about 80% of patients can have facial edema in the morning, and about 30% of patients can have gross hematuria. Some patients can have mild or moderate proteinuria or transient hypertension, and a few severe patients even have congestive heart failure.

In clinical diagnosis, acute nephritis syndrome with a transient decrease of serum C3 occurred 1–3 weeks after streptococcal infection so that clinical diagnosis can be considered. If necessary, a renal biopsy can be performed to make a definite diagnosis.

In clinical treatment, supportive and symptomatic treatment are the primary methods, including bed rest, salt restriction, blood pressure reduction, diuresis, and swelling reduction, etc. When there is an infection, anti-infection treatment can be carried out. Acute nephritis is a self-limiting disease, and in most cases there is a good prognosis. However, there are still a few patients getting worse or becoming "chronic". Early intervention of TCM has a positive effect on relieving edema, hematuria, and sore throat and improving clinical prognosis.

TCM doctors have observed that most patients with acute nephritis will soon have facial and lower limb edema, which belongs to the category of "edema". Moreover, "yang edema" is used to describe its rapid onset. In etiology and pathogenesis, it is considered that its onset is mainly related to exogenous wind pathogen or internal invasion of sore toxin.

In TCM clinical treatment, methods of scattering wind, clearing heat, ventilating lung qi, removing toxicity and diuresis are often used. The classic prescriptions of TCM such as Yuebijiazhu Decoction and Mahuang Lianqiao Chixiaodou Decoction are commonly used.

Yuebijiazhu Decoction is a classic prescription created by Zhang Zhongjing. It is composed of Mahuang (Ephedrae Herba), Shengshigao (Gypsum Fibrosum), Baizhu (Atractylodis Macrocephalae Rhizoma), Shengjiang (Zingiberis Rhizoma Recens), Dazao (Jujubae Fructus) and Gancao (Glycyrrhizae Radix et Rhizoma). It can scatter wind and clear heat, and ventilate lung qi and move water. When acute nephritis edema occurs very rapidly, facial edema firstly appears and then leads to swelling of limbs and body, especially accompanied by fever, aversion to cold, sore limbs, sore throat, and other cold symptoms; for this condition, Yuebijiazhu Decoction is the most suitable.

Mahuang Lianqiao Chixiaodou Decoction was also created by the medical sage Zhang Zhongjing. It is composed of Mahuang (Ephedrae Herba), Lianqiao (Forsythiae Fructus), Chixiaodou (Semen Phaseoli), Xingren (Armeniacae Semen Amarum), Shengzibaipi (Cortex Catalpae), Shengjiang (Zingiberis Rhizoma Recens), Dazao (Jujubae Fructus) and Gancao (Glycyrrhizae Radix et Rhizoma). It can ventilate lung qi and remove toxicity, and promote diuresis and remove edema. This prescription is especially suitable for acute nephritis edema secondary to infectious skin diseases such as impetigo. This prescription can be used when the patient has an acute onset of edema, accompanied by skin sores, small urine volume with red color, fear of wind, fever, red tongue, thin yellow fur, and floating and rapid pulse.

When acute nephritis persists and becomes "chronic", edema may not subside. TCM refers to this lingering edema as "yin edema". In the treatment, supplementing methods are often used, such as invigorating the spleen, tonifying the kidney, warming yang and diuresis, and classic prescriptions of TCM such as

Shipi Beverage, Zhenwu Decoction, and Jingui Shenqi Pill, which have certain curative effects.

2 IgA nephropathy

IgA nephropathy is the most common primary glomerular disease in the world, accounting for 15%–40% of primary glomerular diseases in Europe and Asia. It is also a critical cause of end-stage renal disease. IgA nephropathy can occur at any age, especially in men aged 20–30.

In clinical manifestations, the onset of IgA nephropathy is hidden, often showing asymptomatic hematuria or proteinuria. Some patients may show hypertension, nephrotic syndrome, and renal function damage to varying degrees.

In clinical diagnosis, if microscopic hematuria and proteinuria related to upper respiratory tract infection are found, IgA nephropathy should be considered. Moreover, renal biopsy and immunopathological examination should be performed to make a precise diagnosis.

In clinical treatment, patients with simple microscopic hematuria do not need treatment, but need regular reexamination; for patients with recurrent gross hematuria after infection, non-nephrotoxic medicines should be actively used to resist infection; for patients with proteinuria or hypertension with proteinuria, ARB/ACEI can be used to control urinary protein and blood pressure to protect renal function and delay disease progression.

The prognosis of IgA nephropathy is not optimistic. The survival rate of patients with kidney disease in 10 years is about 80%, and that in 20 years is about 65%. Some patients have poor treatment effects, and even progress quickly to renal failure. It is found that timely intervention of TCM can relieve discomfort, improve hematuria and proteinuria, and delay the deterioration of kidney function.

In TCM, IgA nephropathy belongs to the categories of "kidney-wind edema" and "edema". The etiology is mainly related to exogenous pathogenic qi and weakness of vital qi. In pathogenesis, pathogen invades the throat, and the human body is deficient in vital qi. So, the body can't resist pathogen, and pathogen invades the kidney deeply, causing the disease.

In clinical treatment, the classic prescriptions Fangji Huangqi Decoction and Chinese patent medicine Huangkui Capsule are widely used in clinical practice. Fangji Huangqi Decoction comes from the *Treatise on Cold Pathogenic Diseases* written by Zhang Zhongjing. It is composed of Fangji (Stephaniae Tetrandrae Radix), Huangqi (Astragali Radix), Baizhu (Atractylodis Macrocephalae Rhizoma), Gancao (Glycyrrhizae Radix et Rhizoma), Shengjiang (Zingiberis Rhizoma Recens) and Dazao (Jujubae Fructus). It has the effects of benefiting qi and dispelling pathogenic wind, and invigorating the spleen and diuresis. Clinically, it is often used to treat IgA nephropathy accompanied by easy sweating, fear of wind, eyelid or lower limb edema and limb joint pain. Modern studies have found that this prescription can alleviate the inflammatory reaction of mesangial cells and reduce the proliferation of mesangial cells and the deposition of extramural matrix, delaying the progression of IgA nephropathy.

Huangkui Capsule is a Chinese patent medicine developed in China for treating chronic kidney diseases such as IgA nephropathy. It is especially suitable for chronic kidney disease patients with a damp-heat syndrome such as edema, low back pain, proteinuria, hematuria, and yellow greasy tongue fur. The primary component of Huangkui Capsule is *Abelmoschus corolla*, a traditional medicinal plant in China. According to the *Compendium of Materia Medica*, *Abelmoschus corolla* has the functions of clearing heat and promoting diuresis, and removing toxicity and removing edema. Since Huangkui Capsule was put on the market, more than 15,000 patients with chronic kidney disease have participated in related clinical research, and its efficacy and safety have been recognized by doctors. Especially the randomized, controlled, double-blind, and multicenter clinical trial on the effectiveness and safety of Huangkui Capsule in treating primary glomerular diseases led by Academician Chen Xiangmei of the Chinese Academy of Engineering, a total of 414 patients with primary glomerular diseases were included. Compared with losartan, the 24-hour urinary protein decline rate of Huangkui Capsule was significantly better than that of losartan after 24 weeks of intervention. Moreover, no severe adverse reactions occurred. This achievement, published in *American Journal of Kidney Diseases*, is the high-level evidence-based evidence of nephropathy in Chinese patent medicine. The contents of Huangkui Capsule are brown powders, which taste slightly sweet and bitter. The administration method is 5 capsules each time, 3 times daily, and 8 weeks is a course of treatment.

References

ZHANG L, LI P, XING C Y, et al. Efficacy and safety of Abelmoschus manihot for primary glomerular disease: a prospective, multicenter randomized controlled clinical trial[J]. Am J Kidney Dis, 2014, 64 (1): 57-65.

3 Chronic renal failure

You may have heard that some people need "dialysis" or "kidney transplant" because of chronic renal failure, but you do not know much about chronic renal failure. Chronic renal failure is a major public health problem faced by all countries in the world. It is the common outcome of all kinds of chronic kidney diseases progressing to the later stage. Currently, chronic kidney disease is divided into 5 stages internationally, and chronic renal failure represents the part of chronic kidney disease in which the glomerular filtration rate drops to the decompensation stage, mainly in the fourth to fifth stages.

In etiology, the primary causes of chronic renal failure include diabetic nephropathy, hypertensive renal arteriosclerosis, primary or secondary glomerular diseases, and so on. Hypertension, hyperglycemia, hyperlipidemia, proteinuria, hypoproteinemia, smoking, and the use of nephrotoxic medicines are all critical risk factors for the progression of chronic kidney disease to chronic renal failure.

In clinical symptoms, chronic renal failure is often manifested as edema, fatigue, soreness of the waist, nocturia, and so on. In addition, when cardiovascular, respiratory, digestive, and other systems are involved, it will also show discomforts such as dyspnea, shortness of breath, nausea and vomiting.

In clinical diagnosis, the diagnosis is mainly based on medical history, clinical manifestations, and renal function examination.

In clinical treatment, it includes controlling blood pressure, blood sugar and proteinuria, correcting acidosis and water and electrolyte disorders, correcting anemia, hypocalcemia, and hyperlipidemia, as well as preventing complications such as infection, and dialysis treatment. Clinically, some patients choose integrated traditional Chinese and Western medicine treatment when they have chronic renal insufficiency, which is beneficial to improve symptoms, protect renal function and delay the occurrence of end-stage renal disease.

In TCM, chronic renal failure belongs to the category of "anuria and vomiting". In etiology, it is mainly related to deficiency of yin and yang and qi and blood, blood stasis, turbid phlegm and internal stagnation of water-poison. In pathogenesis, long-term deficient vital qi fails to resist pathogen, and pathogenic toxin invades the kidney, leading to stagnant blockade of kidney collateral, disorder of water passages, and dysfunction of qi transformation, and then renal failure occurs.

In clinical treatment, the therapeutic effects of Dahuang (Rhei Radix et Rhizoma), Huangqi (Astragali Radix), and other single Chinese medicinals on chronic renal failure have been gradually clarified. Chinese patent medicine Niaoduqing Granule composed of Dahuang and Huangqi has been widely used in chronic renal failure because of its reliable curative effect and safety.

Dahuang is the dry root and rhizome of Polygonaceae plants *Rheum palmatum* L., *Rheum tanguticum* Maxim. ex Balf., and *Rheum officinale* Baill. It tastes bitter and cold, and belongs to spleen, stomach, large intestine, liver, and pericardium meridians. It has the effects of attacking accumulation by drastic purgation, clearing heat and removing toxicity, and promoting diuresis and removing jaundice, etc. Modern pharmacological studies have found that rhein, and other active ingredients in Dahuang can inhibit renal interstitial fibrosis and glomerular fibrosis and sclerosis, protect tissue cells, and improve microcirculation and renal function. Huangqi is the dried root of the *Astragalus membranaceus* (Fisch.) Bge. var. *mongholicus* (Bge.) Hsiao or *Astragalus membranaceus* (Fisch.) Bge. It is sweet in taste, slightly warm in nature, and belongs to spleen and lung meridians. It has the effects of diuresis and removing edema, expressing toxin and promoting granulation, benefiting qi and raising yang, and invigorating qi for consolidating superficies, etc. Astragaloside IV, the active component in Huangqi, can improve renal microcirculation and has anti-fibrosis and potential anti-inflammatory effects on chronic renal failure.

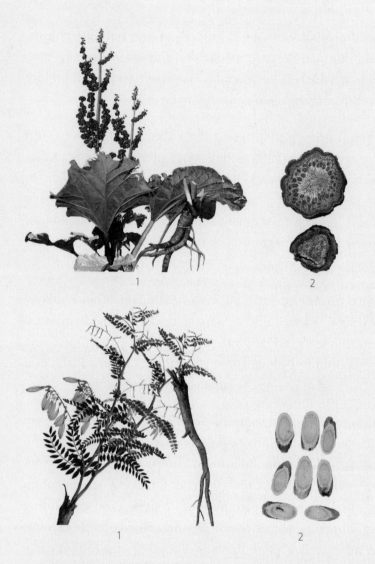

Dahuang
1. Source plant;
2. Decoction pieces.

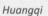

Huangqi
1. Source plant;
2. decoction pieces.

Niaoduqing Granule is composed of Dahuang (Rhei Radix et Rhizoma), Huangqi (Astragali Radix), Gancao (Glycyrrhizae Radix et Rhizoma), Fuling (Poria), Baizhu (Atractylodis Macrocephalae Rhizoma), Heshouwu (Polygoni Multiflori Radix), Chuanxiong (Chuanxiong Rhizoma), Juhua (Chrysanthemi Flos), Danshen (Salviae Miltiorrhizae Radix et Rhizoma) and Banxia (Pinelliae Rhizoma), and other Chinese medicinals. It has the effects of unblocking the bowels and directing the turbid downward, invigorating spleen and promoting diuresis, and promoting blood circulation for removing blood stasis. For patients with chronic renal failure, this medicine can not only reduce creatinine and urea nitrogen and improve renal function, but also improve anemia, hypocalcemia and hyperlipidemia caused by chronic renal failure. Now it has been selected as a "strongly recommended" Chinese patent medicine for treating chronic renal failure in the *Clinical Application Guidelines for Treating Dominant Diseases with Chinese Patent Medicine* in China. The dosage specification of Chinese patent medicine Niaoduqing Granule is 5 g per bag. The administration method is to take them with warm boiled water. It is worth noting that its administration method is unique, requiring patients to take it 4 times daily, 1 bag at 6:00, 12:00 and 18:00, and 2 bags at 22:00.

In addition to oral medicine, acupuncture, moxibustion, acupoint application, enema with Chinese medicinals, and other means can also be used to comprehensively intervene in chronic renal failure, which plays a certain role in relieving edema, and other symptoms of patients and improving their quality of life.

4 Urinary tract infection

Many people have experienced discomforts such as frequent urination, urgent urination, and painful urination, and some people are even accompanied by fever, shivering, low back pain, and other symptoms, which are mainly caused by urinary tract infection. Urinary tract infection is a common infectious disease caused by the growth and reproduction of pathogenic microorganisms in the urinary tract, which affects about 130 million–175 million people every year in the world.

In etiology, this disease is related to pathogens such as bacteria, fungi and mycoplasma. Among them, the most common pathogen is Gram-negative bacilli represented by *Escherichia coli*, accounting for 75%–90% of simple urinary tract infection.

In clinical manifestations, patients often have bladder irritation signs, mainly including frequent micturition, urgent micturition, and painful micturition, and some also have dysuria and turbid urine. If acute pyelonephritis occurs, fever, shivering, headache, and low back pain may also occur.

In clinical diagnosis, besides the clinical manifestations of urinary tract infection, urine routine, bacterial smear, and bacterial culture should be carried out to identify pathogenic bacteria.

With the development of diagnostic methods and the wide use of antibiotics, most patients with urinary tract infection can thoroughly recover after active and reasonable anti-infection treatment. However, in some patients, due to abnormal urinary system structure or low immunity, the infection can not be well controlled. The control with Western medicine alone is not ideal, so it is hoped to combine Chinese medicinals to reduce the frequency of attacks.

In TCM, urinary tract infection belongs to the category of "strangury", which is located in the kidney and bladder. In etiology, it is related to physical weakness and overstrain and exogenous dampness-heat toxin pathogen. In pathogenesis, it is related to the dampness-heat amassment in the lower jiao, disorder of qi transformation of kidney and bladder.

In clinical treatment, classic prescriptions of TCM such as Danggui Beimu Kushen Pill and Bazheng Powder and Chinese patent medicine such as Sanjin Tablet are commonly used. Danggui Beimu Kushen Pill comes from the book *Synopsis of Golden Chamber* written by Zhang Zhongjing. This prescription consists of Danggui (Angelicae Sinensis Radix), Beimu (Bulbus Fritillariae) and Kushen (Sophorae Flavescentis Radix), which are ground into powder in the same proportion, and then blended with honey to make pills with the functions of clearing heat and diuresis, and nourishing blood for tranquilizing fetus to prevent miscarriage. According to the original records, Zhang Zhongjing used this prescription to treat urinary tract infection during pregnancy. In modern clinical application, as long as urinary tract infection has such dampness-heat signs as painful urination, yellow urine, dry stool, red tongue with greasy yellow fur, rapid and slippery pulse, it can be flexibly used for treatment.

Bazheng Powder, recorded in *Prescriptions of the Bureau of Taiping People's Welfare Pharmacy* in the Song Dynasty, is composed of 8 Chinese medicinals, including Cheqianzi (Plantaginis Semen), Qumai (Dianthi Herba), Bianxu (Herba Polygoni Avicularis), Huashi (Talcum), Zhizi (Gardeniae Fructus), Gancao (Glycyrrhizae Radix et Rhizoma), Mutong (Akebiae Caulis) and Dahuang (Rhei Radix et Rhizoma). It has been a famous prescription for treating urinary tract infection since ancient times. It has the effects of clearing heat and removing toxicity, and promoting diuresis and freeing strangury. Bazheng Powder is suitable for patients with acute urinary tract infection with frequent micturition, urgent micturition, and painful micturition, accompanied by turbid urine, acute pain in lower abdomen, thirst, red tongue, greasy yellow fur, and slippery and rapid pulse. Chinese patent medicine Bazheng Mixture, developed from the basic prescription of Bazheng Powder, has been put into clinical use. Its dosage specification is 150 ml or 200 ml per bottle. The administration method is 15–20 ml per oral use, 3 times daily.

Sanjin Tablet has the effects of clearing heat and removing toxicity and promoting diuresis, and freeing strangury. It is a common Chinese patent medicine for treating urinary tract infection. It is mainly composed of Jinyinggen (Rosae Laevigatae Radix), Baqia (Smilacis Chinae Rhizoma), Yangkaikou (Akebiae Caulis), Jinshateng (Lygodii Herba), Jixuecao (Centellae Herba), and other Chinese medicinals. It is especially suitable for patients with urinary tract infection with apparent dampness-heat in lower jiao, such as frequent urination, urgent urination, painful urination, short and red urine, dysphoria with feverish sensation, a bitter taste, red tongue, yellow and greasy fur, and slippery and rapid pulse. A meta-analysis study involving 8 randomized controlled trials, including 790 patients with urinary tract infections, found that Sanjin Tablet has the same curative effect as antibiotics such as levofloxacin, and the combination of Sanjin Tablet and antibiotics can improve the cure rate, total effective rate, and bacterial clearance rate, and reduce the recurrence rate of infection. Sanjin Tablet has two specifications, with a weight of 0.18 g for small tablets and 0.29 g for big tablets. The method is oral administration, with 5 small tablets or 3 big tablets each time, both 3–4 times a day.

References

LYU J, XIE Y, SUN M, et al. Sanjin tablet combined with antibiotics for treating patients with acute lower urinary tract infections: a meta-analysis and GRADE evidence profile [J]. Exp Ther Med, 2020, 19 (1): 683-695.

5 Urinary incontinence

Urinary incontinence refers to the phenomenon that the pressure in the bladder exceeds the urethral resistance during the urine storage period, which is called "unable to hold urine" and is often dubbed as "adults' emotions getting out of control". For patients, this is a very shameful thing, which often seriously affects their physical and mental health and social communication. However, this shameful disease has plagued nearly 2 billion people worldwide. The incidence of urinary incontinence in women is significantly higher than that in men. In China, about one-third of women suffer from this problem, and about 7% of them have apparent urinary incontinence.

In clinical manifestations, patients mainly show that urine flows out uncontrollably when coughing, sneezing, laughing, exercising or carrying heavy objects. When they are in a hurry to get to the toilet, or even when they drink water, or hear the sound of running water, or get nervous, they cannot control urination. Some patients sometimes have symptoms such as hematuria, dysuria or pelvic pain.

Clinically, the diagnosis can be made according to the above typical clinical manifestations, combined with relevant obstetric and gynecological history and physical examination.

In clinical treatment, pelvic floor muscle training represented by Kegel exercise can be carried out to improve pelvic floor function and urethral stability. Drugs such as duloxetine, estrogen, and other medicines can also be used for treatment, or surgical treatment such as a mid-urethral sling surgery. In order to avoid the trauma caused by surgical treatment, many patients often prefer to choose non-surgical treatment such as drug therapy and rehabilitation training.

In TCM, urinary incontinence belongs to the category of "enuresis" and "uncontrolled urination". The disease is located in bladder and kidney, and its etiology is related to physical weakness due to long-term illness and excessive delivery. In pathogenesis, it is due to physical weakness and overstrain, loss of kidney qi due to excessive delivery, and dysfunction of bladder due to non-consolidation of kidney qi. So, urination is uncontrolled.

In clinical treatment, the classic prescriptions of TCM represented by Jingui Shenqi Pill and acupuncture are often used for treatment. Jingui Shenqi Pill is a classic prescription created by Zhang Zhongjing. It is composed of 8 Chinese medicinals: Guizhi (Cinnamomi Ramulus), Fuzi (Aconiti Lateralis Radix Praeparata), Shengdihuang (Rehmanniae Radix), Shanyao (Dioscoreae Rhizoma), Shanzhuyu (Corni Fructus), Zexie (Alismatis Rhizoma), Fuling (Poria) and

Mudanpi (Moutan Cortex), and is the representative prescription for warming and tonifying kidney yang. This prescription can warm kidney yang, and supplement kidney essence, making kidney qi sufficient and the bladder function normal. It is especially suitable for urinary incontinence patients with sore waist and knees, fear of cold, cold limbs, pale tongue, and deep and weak pulse. This prescription has been made into Chinese patent medicine and put into the market. Generally, 360 pills are contained in each bottle. The administration method is oral. Twenty-five pills are to be taken each time and twice daily, but it should be noted that pregnant women should not take it.

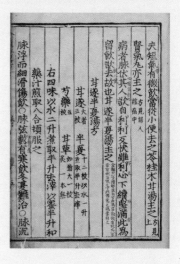

The article of Shenqi Pill

The treatment method of TCM, represented by acupuncture, also shows unique clinical advantages in treating female urinary incontinence, and has been widely used in the clinic. In 2017, *The Journal of the American Medical Association* (JAMA), an international top medical journal, published a randomized clinical trial on the efficacy of electroacupuncture on urine leakage of female stress urinary incontinence, which was completed by Professor Liu Baoyan of China Academy of Chinese Medical Sciences and chief physician Liu Zhishun of Guang'anmen Hospital. It has been found that electroacupuncture at Zhōngliáo (BL33) and Huìyáng (BL35) in the lumbosacral region, 3 times a week for a total of 6 weeks, can effectively relieve female stress urinary incontinence, and the curative effect is lasting with few adverse reactions, which brings good news to the majority of urinary incontinence patients.

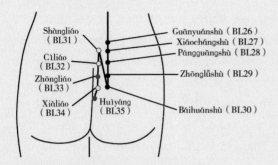

Shàngliáo (BL31)
Cìliáo (BL32)
Zhōngliáo (BL33)
Xiàliáo (BL34)
Huìyáng (BL35)
Guānyuánshù (BL26)
Xiǎochángshù (BL27)
Pángguāngshù (BL28)
Zhōnglǚshù (BL29)
Báihuánshù (BL30)

Zhōngliáo (BL33) and
Huìyáng (BL35)

References

LIU Z S, LIU Y, XU H F, et al. Effect of electroacupuncture on urinary leakage among women with stress urinary incontinence: a randomized clinical trial[J]. JAMA, 2017, 317 (24): 2493-2501.

Section 5
Blood System Diseases

| Overview of blood system diseases

Hematological diseases are diseases originating from the hematopoietic system or diseases affecting the hematopoietic system with abnormal blood changes. The hematopoietic system consists of blood, bone marrow, monocyte-macrophage system, and lymphoid tissue. All diseases involving the pathophysiology of the hematopoietic system and taking it as the primary manifestation belong to the category of hematological diseases. Clinical common blood system diseases include anemia, leukopenia and agranulocytosis, hypersplenism, leukemia, hemophilia, purpura, and so on.

In clinical treatment, it mainly includes radiotherapy and chemotherapy, hematopoietic stem cell and bone marrow transplantation, splenectomy, and so on. However, due to the particularity of blood, most hematological diseases have problems such as a long course of the disease, many complications, easy recurrence, and a low control rate. Infection, hemorrhage, coagulation dysfunction, thrombocytosis after splenectomy, decreased immune system function, thrombus, and other sequelae seriously affect the quality of life.

In TCM, blood system diseases belong to the category of "consumptive disease". In recent years, with the clinical evidence of the arsenic treatment for leukemia published in the *New England Journal of Medicine*, the advantages of TCM in treating hematological diseases have gradually attracted global attention. In addition to arsenic, a large number of clinical evidences have been gradually revealed, such as Datusizi Beverage for aplastic anemia, Qinghuang Powder for chronic myeloid leukemia and myelodysplastic syndrome, and Compound Huangdai Tablet for acute promyelocytic leukemia. In this section, we will focus on anemia, aplastic anemia, leukopenia, and leukemia, elaborating the advantages and schemes of clinical diagnosis and treatment of TCM.

‖ Treatises on blood system diseases

1 Anemia

In daily life, people often feel weak, with a pale and terrible complexion, especially women. Most people around you will say: Are you anemic? It can be seen that the incidence of anemia in the population is not low. Let us take a closer look at this anemia we seem familiar with.

Anemia means that the number of red blood cells and hemoglobin content per unit volume of blood is lower than normal. Anemia can be diagnosed according to the amount of hemoglobin. For men, anemia can be diagnosed if hemoglobin is lower than 120 g/L, and for women, anemia can be diagnosed if hemoglobin is lower than 110 g/L. According to the amount of hemoglobin, anemia can generally be divided into 3 levels: mild, moderate, and severe. Hemoglobin at 90–110/120 g/L can be diagnosed as mild anemia. When hemoglobin is 60–90 g/L, moderate anemia can be diagnosed. When hemoglobin is lower than 60g/L, severe anemia can be diagnosed.

There are many causes of anemia, including iron deficiency, hemorrhage, hemolysis, hematopoietic dysfunction, and so on. In clinical symptoms, the symptoms are dizziness, fatigue, insomnia, dreaminess, memory loss, pale skin, eyelids, etc. The primary distinguishing features are pale skin, nails, and eyelids. Among anemia, iron deficiency anemia is the most common.

Clinical treatment mainly includes symptomatic treatment of blood transfusion and etiological treatment such as iron supplement and folic acid. However, clinically, patients often suffer from dizziness repeatedly, and their symptoms are not relieved obviously, so they turn to TCM for treatment.

In TCM, anemia belongs to the categories of "blood deficiency" and "consumptive disease". In pathogenesis, anemia belongs to deficiency syndrome, mainly characterized by deficiency of spleen qi and marrow depletion due to kidney deficiency. According to TCM, spleen and stomach are the sources of generation and transformation of qi and blood, and the generation of blood is most closely related to spleen. Eating disorders, overstrain, and physical weakness for long-term illness can all damage the function of spleen and stomach, leading to anemia. In clinical practice, the classic prescriptions Danggui Buxue Decoction and Guipi Decoction are the most commonly used.

Danggui Buxue Decoction comes from Li Dongyuan, a famous doctor in the Jin and Yuan Dynasties. It is composed of Huangqi (Astragali Radix) for invigorating qi and Danggui (Angelicae Sinensis Radix) for enriching the blood with the dosage ratio of 5 : 1. In the prescription, Huangqi is used to tonify spleen and lung qi, and Danggui is used to enrich blood and nourish blood, which is especially suitable for anemia patients with deficiency of qi and blood. This kind of patient can manifest as dizziness, burnout and fatigue when moving, palpitation, shortness of breath, tender and pale tongue, thin white fur, and deep and weak pulse. In ancient times, Danggui Buxue Decoction was used as the basic prescription, and many good prescriptions for invigorating qi and enriching the blood were made. Shengyu Decoction is an example, including Huangqi (Astragali Radix), Renshen (Ginseng Radix et Rhizoma), Danggui (Angelicae Sinensis Radix), Dihuang (Rehmanniae Radix), Baishao (Paeoniae Radix Alba) and Chuanxiong (Chuanxiong Rhizoma), which can treat patients with blood loss and anemia.

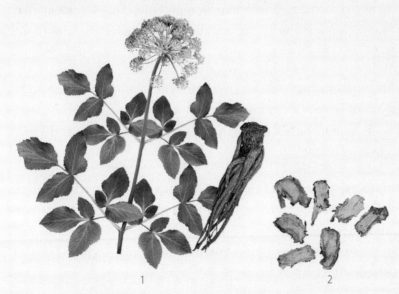

Danggui
1. Source plant;
2. decoction pieces.

Guipi Decoction comes from *Re-ordering Yan's Jisheng Prescription*, which is composed of Renshen (Ginseng Radix et Rhizoma), Baizhu (Atractylodis Macrocephalae Rhizoma), Fuling (Poria), Huangqi (Astragali Radix), Zhigancao (Glycyrrhizae Radix et Rhizoma Praeparata cum Melle), Danggui (Angelicae

Sinensis Radix), Yuanzhi (Polygalae Radix), Suanzaoren (Ziziphi Spinosae Semen), Longyanrou (Longan Arillus), Muxiang (Aucklandiae Radix) and Dazao (Jujubae Fructus). This prescription has the effects of invigorating qi and nourishing blood, and invigorating the spleen and heart. It is especially suitable for patients with syndrome of blood deficiency of heart and spleen. The clinical manifestations are sallow complexion, burnout, spirit fatigue, spontaneous sweating, palpitation, shortness of breath, dizziness, loss of appetite, nausea, and vomiting, abdominal pain and diarrhea, pale and enlarged tongue and thready and weak pulse. Modern pharmacological studies have found that this prescription can enhance hematopoietic function. Nowadays, the Chinese patent medicine Guipi Pill, commonly used in the clinic, comes from the original prescription of Guipi Decoction, and the dosage is 9 g each time, 3 times daily.

2 Aplastic anemia

Aplastic anemia is a kind of bone marrow failure syndrome, simply the decline in bone marrow hematopoietic function. The annual incidence of aplastic anemia in China is 0.74/100,000. The patient has pancytopenia, and the clinical manifestation is anemia, or combined with infection and bleeding. The incidence of this disease is mainly among young and middle-aged population, with more males than females.

In pathogenesis, the etiology of acquired aplastic anemia is unclear at present, and occupational exposure to benzene and its derivatives is the clearest etiology. Others such as anti-tumor medicines, ionizing radiation, and virus infection have also been reported.

In clinical symptoms, severe aplastic anemia starts quickly and develops rapidly, with bleeding, infection, and fever as the first symptoms. This disease has a poor prognosis and high mortality. The onset and development of non-severe aplastic anemia are slow, with primary anemia manifestations such as fatigue, palpitation, and pale complexion.

In clinical treatment, Western medicine often takes immunosuppressant, bone marrow transplantation, androgen stimulating bone marrow hematopoiesis, and other supportive therapies such as infection control and component blood transfusion as the primary treatment means. However, immunosuppressants may decrease immune system function, and are easily complicated with infection. They have certain hepatorenal toxicity; bone marrow transplantation is suitable for a narrow population; androgen therapy has a certain degree of masculinity and hepatotoxicity. Many patients with aplastic anemia will seek aggressive treatment from TCM. TCM has certain advantages in treating chronic aplastic anemia, which can reduce complications, such as infection, skin petechia, gingival bleeding, etc., and regulate the immune system, reducing adverse reactions of Western medicine and improving patients' quality of life.

In TCM, aplastic anemia belongs to the categories of "consumptive disease with syndrome of heat obstructing heart and lung", "consumptive disease with syndrome of kidney essence insufficiency", and "consumptive disease". In etiology, this disease is mainly caused by pathogenic toxin direct attacking and damaging marrow, which includes medicines, radiation, and so on. In pathogenesis, this disease is based on marrow depletion and essence deficiency as the root cause, and deficiency of qi and blood as manifestation.

Clinically, the classic prescription Zhigancao Decoction and Huangqi Injection are commonly used in the clinic. Zhigancao Decoction comes from *Treatise on Cold Pathogenic Diseases*, which is composed of Zhigancao (Glycyrrhizae Radix et Rhizoma Praeparata cum Melle), Renshen (Ginseng Radix et Rhizoma), Ganjiang (Zingiberis Rhizoma), Guizhi (Cinnamomi Ramulus), Maidong (Ophiopogonis Radix), Shengdihuang (Rehmanniae Radix), Huomaren (Cannabis Fructus), Ejiao (Asini Corii Colla) and Dazao (Jujubae Fructus). It has the functions of invigorating qi and restoring pulse, and nourishing yin and unblocking yang. Because Zhigancao Decoction can effectively increase the number of blood cells, it is often used to treat various hematopenia caused by bleeding or other reasons, such as aplastic anemia, severe anemia, thrombocytopenia, leukopenia, etc. Modern pharmacological research has shown that Renshen (Ginseng Radix et Rhizoma) and Ejiao (Asini Corii Colla) in the prescription can improve the hematopoietic function of bone marrow, while Zhigancao (Glycyrrhizae Radix et Rhizoma Praeparata cum Melle) and Shengdi (raw Rehmanniae Radix) as sovereign medicine can improve the immunity of the body, and Shengdihuang (Rehmanniae Radix) has some effects on resisting ionizing radiation.

Huangqi Injection, refined from the single Chinese medicinal Huangqi

(Astragali Radix) and sodium bicarbonate, has the functions of invigorating qi to consolidate superficies, invigorating the spleen and tonifying middle jiao, and strengthening vital qi to eliminate pathogenic factor. Pharmacological studies have shown that Huangqi has an apparent effect on stimulating bone marrow hematopoiesis, regulating the immune response bidirectionally, enhancing body resistance, and reducing complications such as infection. Clinically, the dosage and administration is, 2–4 ml once, 1–2 times daily for intramuscular injection, or 10–20 ml once, once daily for intravenous drip.

References

XIONG X J. Traceability of Zhigancao Decoction based on modern pathophysiology and CCU acute and critical cases and its clinical application of cardioversion, sinus conversion, hemostasis, platelet raising and deficiency tonifying [J]. China Journal of Chinese Materia Medica, 2019, 44 (18): 19.

3 Leukopenia

Leukopenia is a condition in which peripheral blood leukocytes are consistently lower than 4×10^9/L. More than half of leukocytes are neutrophils. If the neutrophils in peripheral blood are lower than 2×10^9/L, it is called granulocytopenia.

In etiology, leukopenia is closely related to the direct killing of peripheral leukocytes by tumor radiotherapy and chemotherapy, various medicines such as antipyretic analgesics ibuprofen and aspirin, antithyroid medicines, antibiotics, cardiovascular medicines, infection and immune system diseases, physical and chemical factors, including ionizing radiation, benzene, toluene, etc.

In clinical symptoms, this disease is mainly a chronic process, which may be accompanied by dizziness, fatigue, loss of appetite, low fever, low back pain, etc. If the granulocytes are less than 1×10^9/L, secondary infections such as stomatitis, otitis media, bronchitis, pneumonia, and pyelonephritis may occur.

Clinical treatment includes removing etiology, combining work with rest, proper exercise, controlling infection, glucocorticoids, and medicines to promote granulocyte production. Because some patients have adverse reaction to the treatment such as intolerance to glucocorticoids, and partial symptomatic treatment is prone to relapse and cannot effectively improve the quality of life of patients with leukopenia. Clinically, many patients come to the clinic for TCM treatment.

In TCM, this disease belongs to the category of "insufficiency" and "consumptive disease". In etiology, it is mainly related to being attacked by external pathogen, medicine toxin, insufficiency of congenital endowment, eating disorder, overstrain and internal damage, long-term illness and severe illness. In pathogenesis, this disease is the syndrome of excessive manifestation and deficient root, mainly deficiency of qi and blood and deficiency of spleen and kidney.

Clinically, classic prescription Bazhen Decoction and Chinese patent medicine Diyu Shengbai Tablet are commonly used. Bazhen Decoction comes from *Essentials of Bonesetting*, which is composed of Renshen (Ginseng Radix et Rhizoma), Baizhu (Atractylodis Macrocephalae Rhizoma), Fuling (Poria), Gancao (Glycyrrhizae Radix et Rhizoma), Danggui (Angelicae Sinensis Radix), Shudihuang (Rehmanniae Radix Praeparata), Shaoyao (Paeoniae Radix Alba seu Rubra) and Chuanxiong (Chuanxiong Rhizoma). It contains Sijunzi Decoction for invigorating the spleen and qi and Siwu Decoction for nourishing blood and enriching blood, and is a classic prescription for benefiting qi and blood. Bazhen Decoction is widely used in leukopenia accompanied by shortness of breath, laziness to talk, limb burnout, loss of appetite, and other debilitating symptoms. Modern pharmacological studies have confirmed that Bazhen Decoction can improve immune system ability, promote hematopoietic function and kill tumor cells to some extent. Clinical studies have also found that this prescription can not only be used to improve leukopenia caused by the tumor, radiotherapy and chemotherapy, methimazole, and other reasons, but also effectively improve related clinical symptoms and quality of life.

Diyu Shengbai Tablet is mainly composed of Diyu (Sanguisorbae Radix). Compared with expensive medicines such as leucogen and recombinant human granulocyte stimulating factor, it has the advantages of stable curative effect, low price, and high safety. Currently, it has been widely used in leukopenia caused by radiotherapy and chemotherapy, as well as taking antithyroid medicines such as methimazole and interferon. Modern pharmacological studies have shown that Diyu (Sanguisorbae Radix) can promote the proliferation of bone marrow cells and increase the number of nucleated cells in bone marrow. It can also increase the number of white blood cells, red blood cells, and platelets in peripheral blood, and effectively stop bleeding. The clinical administration method is oral, 2–4 tablets each time, 3 times daily.

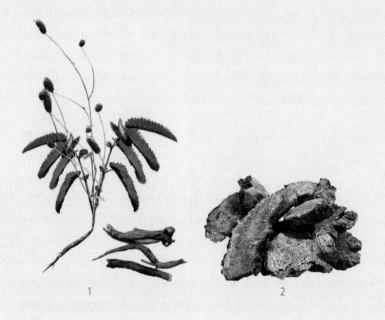

Diyu
1. Source plant;
2. decoction pieces.

4 Leukemia

Leukemia, commonly known as "blood cancer", is a malignant clonal disease of hematopoietic stem cells and belongs to the malignant tumor. In China, the annual incidence of leukemia is increasing year by year.

In pathogenesis, the disease is related to virus infection, ionizing radiation, chemical substances, heredity, and so on. Among them, some anti-tumor medicines are closely related to this disease. The epidemiological investigation found that long-term occupational exposure or daily exposure to benzene and its derivatives, dyes, and hair dyes were critical reasons.

In clinical symptoms, acute leukemia occurs rapidly, often accompanied by high fever, infection, bleeding, anemia, hepatosplenomegaly, skeletal muscle joint pain, nausea, vomiting, etc. Anemia and thrombocytopenia are the most common in laboratory examination, and hyperplasia of bone marrow image is obviously active or hyperactive as the primary basis for its diagnosis. Chronic leukemia is mainly hepatosplenomegaly, and clinical manifestations such as low fever, sweating, and emaciation can also be seen.

In clinical treatment, it is necessary to formulate effective treatment plans in combination with clinical classification and prognosis stratification, which mainly include chemotherapy, radiotherapy, targeted therapy, immunotherapy, stem cell transplantation, and so on. Although chemotherapy is the primary clinical treatment at present, it has severe side effects. This disease is easy to relapse in clinic, and the treatment cost is high, which brings a heavy medical burden to patients.

In TCM, leukemia belongs to the categories of "consumptive disease" "consumptive disease with syndrome of deficient heat", "100-day consumptive disease" and "concretions and accumulation". In pathogenesis, this disease is related to heat-toxin, phlegm coagulation, blood stasis, and deficient vital qi, which are reciprocal causation, forming the syndrome of intermingled deficiency and excess. In recent years, the clinical advantages of TCM in treating leukemia, such as targeted anti-cancer, improvement of symptoms, less toxic and side effects, attenuating toxicity and enhancing effectiveness with the combined use of Chinese and Western medicine, have gradually attracted attention, especially the breakthrough of arsenic trioxide in treating leukemia.

Ailing No.1 Injection is developed from Chinese medicinal—arsenic, and its primary components are arsenic trioxide and arsenite. Studies have shown that a safe remission rate of 91% for acute promyelocytic leukemia 72% for chronic myeloid leukemia, and 70% for lymphoma. Because of its ability to cross the blood-brain barrier, the occurrence of central nervous system leukemia is largely avoided in treatment. No strong toxic reactions and bone marrow suppression were observed in clinic. Some patients had nausea, stomach distension, skin itching, and other reactions, which can disappear after medicine withdrawal or symptomatic treatment. In addition, Ailing No.1 Injection can also promote megakaryocyte proliferation and platelet production. The primary mechanism of arsenic treatment is to induce differentiation and apoptosis of leukemia cells.

It is different from the previous radiotherapy and chemotherapy, which is non-selective and kills all of them regardless of good or bad. The medicine has targeted selectivity to leukemia cells and detours to normal cells, so the curative effect is more accurate and the safety is higher. Based on Ailing No.1 Injection, clinical and basic research on arsenic treatment of leukemia has been carried out in China, and has quickly attracted international attention. Sloan-Ketting and others gave arsenic treatment to 12 patients with recurrent acute promyelocytic leukemia after conventional treatment, and 11 patients got complete remission. After the article was published in *The New England Journal of Medicine*, the clinical efficacy of arsenic in treating leukemia began to be generally accepted internationally.

References

SOIGNET S L, MASLAK P, WANG Z G, et al. Complete remission after treatment of acute promyelocytic leukemia with arsenic trioxide[J]. New England Journal of Medicine, 1998, 339 (19): 1341-1348.

Section 6
Endocrine and Metabolic Diseases

I Overview of endocrine and metabolic diseases

It is often seen that some people will doubt whether they belong to "endocrine disorders" or "metabolic disorders" once they have symptoms such as acne, irregular menstruation, fear of heat and sweating, insomnia, etc. or when they find elevated blood sugar and blood lipid or abnormal hormone levels during physical examination. In fact, such doubts are not unreasonable.

Endocrine system comprises endocrine glands such as the pituitary gland, thyroid gland, and adrenal gland, and endocrine tissues and cells distributed all over the body. Various hormones are produced and secreted into the blood, acting on target organs and tissues, and maintaining normal physiological functions of the human body. There are many kinds of endocrine and metabolic diseases, the most common of which include thyroid diseases such as hyperthyroidism, hypothyroidism and thyroid nodules, diabetes, hyperlipidemia, etc.

In clinical treatment, for patients with hyperfunction, surgical resection and medical treatment can be selected to reduce hormone release from endocrine tumors or hyperplastic tissues; for patients with hypofunction, corresponding exogenous hormones can be supplemented, such as levothyroxine sodium for hypothyroidism. However, we have found that some patients are not satisfied with long-term oral medicine maintenance, including long-term oral levothyroxine, hypoglycemic medicines, lipid-lowering medicines, etc., and some patients also hope for TCM treatment because of adverse reactions after Western medicine treatment.

In recent years, TCM have made continuous progress in the clinical treatment of endocrine and metabolic diseases, and have been increasingly recognized internationally. Endocrine and metabolic diseases belong to the categories of "consumptive disease", "goiter disease", "consumptive thirst", "turbid blood", etc. in TCM. Clinically, TCM has shown certain clinical value in improving thyroid function, reducing thyroid nodules, regulating glucose and lipid metabolism, alleviating diabetic complications, and improving related clinical symptoms. This section will focus on the clinical diagnosis and treatment of hypothyroidism, thyroid nodules, diabetes, and its complications, and dyslipidemia.

‖ Treatises on endocrine and metabolic diseases

1 Hypothyroidism

Hypothyroidism refers to a hypometabolic syndrome caused by the decrease of thyroid hormone levels or thyroid hormone resistance in blood due to various reasons. The etiology is often associated with autoimmune thyroiditis, thyroid surgery injury, and ^{131}I treatment.

In clinical manifestations, early or mild patients may not have specific symptoms. In contrast, typical patients may have symptoms of hypofunction of metabolism and hypoacticity of sympathetic nerves, such as shivering, fatigue, lethargy, memory loss, slow response, hypohidrosis, menstrual disorder, weight gain, edema, etc.

In clinical diagnosis, thyroid-related history, such as operation history and ^{131}I treatment history, should be inquired, combined with clinical manifestations of patients, and serum TSH, TT_4 and FT_4 should be examined.

In clinical treatment, the primary treatment method at present is levothyroxine treatment, and the commonly used medicine is known as "eugenol". The treatment goal is stabilizing serum TSH and thyroid hormone at normal levels. The effect of taking medicine is better, but patients are required to take medicine regularly throughout their life and to review hormone indexes regularly. To a certain extent, there are many inconveniences. TCM has certain clinical value and significance in treating hypothyroidism, and has certain advantages in improving the symptoms related to hypothyroidism.

In TCM, hypothyroidism belongs to the category of "consumptive disease", "edema", and "goiter exhaustion". In etiology, it is closely related to emotions and internal damage, physical weakness and overstrain, diet and environment, and physical factors. In pathogenesis, various factors, such as emotions and internal damage, and physical weakness due to long-term illness, lead to the decline in zang-fu viscera function. Then, a series of "deficient consumption"-based manifestations appear. The most common symptoms of hypothyroidism include fear of cold, fatigue, lethargy, memory loss, slow response, and other systemic symptoms of low metabolism and low sympathetic nerve excitability, which belong to the category of kidney-yang deficiency in TCM.

In clinical treatment, the classic prescriptions Jingui Shenqi Pill and Zhenwu Decoction are often used. In addition, moxibustion, acupuncture, and other external treatments of TCM can also be selected. Jingui Shenqi Pill is a famous prescription created by Zhang Zhongjing. It is composed of 8 Chinese medicinals, including Fuzi (Aconiti Lateralis Radix Praeparata), Guizhi (Cinnamomi Ramulus), Shengdihuang (Rehmanniae Radix), Shanyao (Dioscoreae Rhizoma), Shanzhuyu (Corni Rructus), Zexie (Alismatis Rhizoma), Fuling (Poria) and Mudanpi (Moutan Cortex). It has the effect of warmly invigorating kidney yang. Clinically, it can be used for hypothyroidism patients with kidney-yang deficiency syndrome, such as fear of cold, listlessness, lethargy, soreness and coldness of waist and knees, edema, etc. Jingui Shenqi Pill has been developed into Chinese patent medicine and is widely used in the clinic. Its specification is generally water-honeyed pill, weighing 20 g per 100 pills with 360 pills per bottle. The administration method is to take 20 pills each time, twice a day, but it should be noted that pregnant women should not take it.

Zhenwu Decoction is also a classic prescription created by the medical sage Zhang Zhongjing. It consists of 5 Chinese medicinals: Fuzi (Aconiti Lateralis Radix Praeparata), Fuling (Poria), Baizhu (Atractylodis Macrocephalae Rhizoma), Baishao (Paeoniae Radix Alba), and Shengjiang (Zingiberis Rhizoma Recens). It has the effects of warming yang and promoting urination. It is suitable for hypothyroidism patients with the syndrome of yang deficiency of spleen and kidney and internal stagnation of fluid-dampness. The clinical symptoms of hypothyroidism patients treated with Zhenwu Decoction are often heavier than those of patients with Shenqi Pill syndrome. Based on fear of cold, cold limbs, listlessness and slow response, there are often apparent edema, plump tongue with teeth marks, slow and deep pulse, and other manifestations.

Acupuncture and moxibustion are also methods of treating hypothyroidism in TCM. Stimulates Shènshù (BL23), Píshù (BL20), Guānyuán (CV4) and Zúsānlǐ

(ST36), and other acupoints with tonifying and strengthening effects with acupuncture or moxibustion, which has a certain curative effect on relieving symptoms such as fear of cold, fatigue, listlessness and edema of hypothyroidism patients.

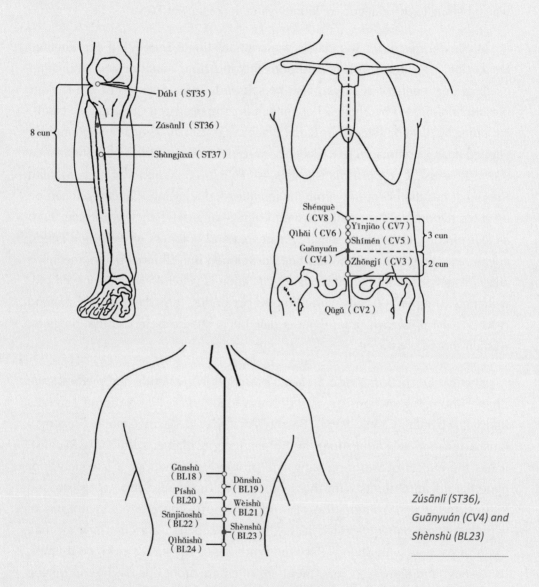

Zúsānlǐ (ST36), Guānyuán (CV4) and Shènshù (BL23)

2 Thyroid nodule

Thyroid nodules are common in the clinic, and about 50% of people can be detected with thyroid nodules by ultrasound. Most nodules are benign adenomatous nodules or cysts, but 5%–10% of nodules are malignant. Many people are always worried about whether thyroid nodules are malignant or will develop into malignant. Its etiology and pathogenesis are still unclear.

In clinical manifestations, most patients with thyroid nodules do not show any clinical symptoms. Some patients may have related symptoms due to hypothyroidism or hyperthyroidism. Some patients with malignant nodules will show cough and short breath due to the compression of trachea by the mass, and dysphagia due to the compression of esophagus.

In clinical diagnosis, it can be comprehensively judged by combining past medical history, clinical manifestations, serum TSH, and other laboratory tests and ultrasound examinations. In addition, ultrasound-guided fine needle aspiration cytology is the gold standard for differentiating benign and malignant nodules, with an accuracy of over 90%, which can be selected when necessary.

In clinical treatment, malignant nodules or nodules with compression symptoms generally need surgical treatment, and nodules with autonomic secretion function can be treated with radioactive iodine. Benign nodules are generally reviewed regularly without unique treatment. Because of its high incidence and malignant transformation possibility, thyroid nodules make many patients suffer from tremendous psychological pressure. They hope to take active treatment to avoid nodule enlargement or malignant transformation, and then seek TCM treatment.

TCM plays a certain role in reducing nodules and improving physique. In TCM, thyroid nodules belong to the category of "goiter" and "phlegm nodule". In etiology, thyroid nodule is mainly related to emotions and internal damage, diet, and inadaptation to the environment, and constitution factors. In pathogenesis, it is mainly related to liver depression and qi stagnation, and intermingled phlegm and qi and static blood in throat.

In clinical treatment, the classic prescriptions Banxia Houpo Decoction, and Xiaoluo Pill are commonly used. Banxia Houpo Decoction comes from *Synopsis of Golden Chamber* written by Zhang Zhongjing. It is composed of 5 Chinese medicinals: Banxia (Pinelliae Rhizoma), Houpo (Magnoliae Officinalis Cortex), Fuling (Poria), Shengjiang (Zingiberis Rhizoma Recens), and Zisuye (Perillae

Folium). This prescription is mainly used to treat "Meiheqi", which is similar to chronic pharyngitis. "Treating different diseases with the same method" is a unique and intelligent theory in TCM, which means that different diseases can be treated in the same way on the condition that different diseases have the same or similar pathogenesis. Because this prescription has the effects of activating qi and resolving hard mass and lowering adverse qi, and eliminating phlegm, it fits the pathogenesis of qi stagnation, phlegm coagulation, and blood stasis of thyroid nodules. It is now widely used to treat thyroid nodules. It should be noted that the medicinals of Banxia Houpo Decoction tend to be warm and dry, which is easy to consume yin fluid of the human body, and is not suitable for patients with yin deficiency such as dry throat and mouth, red tongue and yellow fur, and thready and rapid pulse.

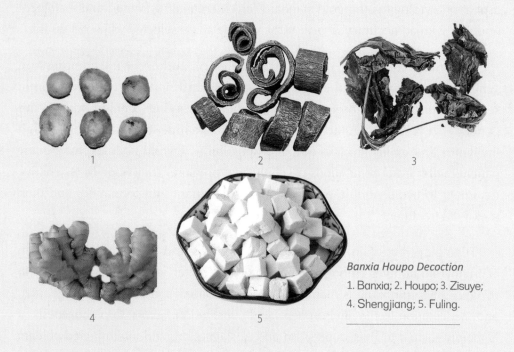

Banxia Houpo Decoction
1. Banxia; 2. Houpo; 3. Zisuye;
4. Shengjiang; 5. Fuling.

Xiaoluo Pill is recorded in the *Medical Revelations* written by Cheng Guopeng, a doctor in the Qing Dynasty. It is composed of Xuanshen (Scrophulariae Radix), Muli (Ostreae Concha), and Beimu (Bulbus Fritillaria). It has the effects of clearing heat and eliminating phlegm, and softening and resolving hard mass. Unlike Banxia Houpo Decoction, Xiaoluo Pill treats nodules caused by liver depression transforming into fire, burning thin fluids into phlegm.

Patients may be accompanied by the symptoms of internal retention of phlegm-heat such as a bitter taste, dry throat, dysphoria with feverish sensation, red tongue with yellow or yellow greasy fur, and stringy or slippery and rapid pulse. Neixiao Luoli Pill, a Chinese patent medicine developed based on Xiaoluo Pill, can clear heat and nourish yin, and eliminate phlegm and soften hard mass, and is used to treat thyroid nodules, and other diseases.

3 Dyslipidemia

In the clinic we often see some elderly people with coronary heart disease particularly concerned about their blood lipid levels, and worried that dyslipidemia will aggravate coronary artery disease and induce angina pectoris, and myocardial infarction. Dyslipidemia generally refers to the increase of cholesterol, triglyceride and low-density lipoprotein cholesterol levels and the decrease of high-density lipoprotein cholesterol levels in serum. The proportion of dyslipidemia in Chinese adults is as high as 40.4%, which is a critical risk factor for cardiovascular and cerebrovascular diseases.

In etiology, most dyslipidemia is caused by genetic defects and environmental factors, so dyslipidemia has certain familial aggregation. Some are caused by hypothyroidism, nephrotic syndrome or taking certain medicines.

In clinical manifestations, lipid deposition under the endothelium of blood vessels will cause atherosclerosis, and some patients will have "xanthoma", "corneal ring" or fundus diseases due to local lipid deposition.

In clinical diagnosis, laboratory serum examination can help us to know the lipid levels for diagnosis. It should be noted that patients should fast for more than 12 hours before blood lipid examination, and the last meal should be light.

In clinical treatment, statins, such as atorvastatin and rosuvastatin, are the first choice for lipid regulation. Of course, comprehensive interventions such as proper diet, weight loss, smoking cessation, and alcohol restriction or medication are also needed.

In TCM, dyslipidemia belongs to the categories of "phlegm-turbidity", "turbid blood" and "lazyitis". In etiology, it is mainly related to deficiency of spleen and kidney, fat and sweet diet, improper work and rest, blockade of phlegm-turbidity, and congenital endowment. In pathogenesis, TCM thinks that "being diligent is strong, and being lazy is sick". Modern people eat more fat and sweet food but lack exercise. If the congenital endowment is insufficient, there is dysfunction of spleen in transportation, dysfunction of kidney in qi transformation, and internal generation of phlegm-turbidity, flowing into the blood, which will lead to abnormal blood lipid.

In TCM treatment, Gegen Qinlian Decoction and Chinese patent medicine Xuezhikang Capsule are often selected. Gegen Qinlian Decoction comes from *Treatise on Cold Pathogenic Diseases* written by Zhang Zhongjing. It is composed of 4 Chinese medicinals: Gegen (Puerariae Lobatae Radix), Huangqin (Scutellariae Radix), Huanglian (Coptidis Rhizoma), and Gancao (Glycyrrhizae Radix et Rhizoma). It has the function of resolving the superficies and clearing the interior. This prescription was initially used to treat diarrhea caused by pathogenic qi penetrating inward due to non-recovery of cold. Modern studies have found that Gegen (Puerariae Lobatae Radix), Huanglian (Coptidis Rhizoma), and Huangqin (Scutellariae Radix) in Gegen Qinlian Decoction have good effects on reducing blood lipid. This prescription is especially suitable for patients with dyslipidemia accompanied by a bitter taste, polydipsia, diarrhea, red tongue, greasy yellow fur, and slippery and rapid pulse.

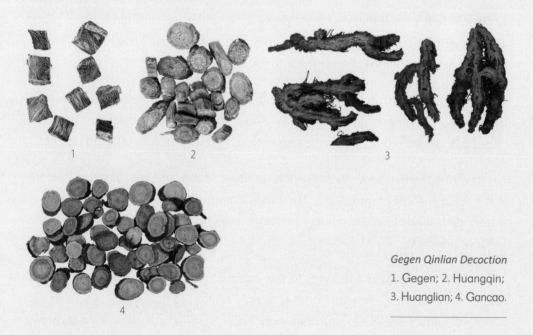

Gegen Qinlian Decoction
1. Gegen; 2. Huangqin;
3. Huanglian; 4. Gancao.

Hongqu is a kind of Chinese medicinal, made by parasitizing *Monascus purpureus* on japonica rice. It has the effects of promoting digestion and harmonizing the stomach, promoting blood circulation to relieve pain and invigorating the spleen. Xuezhikang Capsule is a Chinese patent medicine for regulating blood lipid developed for hyperlipidemia. It is made of indica rice inoculated with unique *Monascus purpureus*, and contains 13 natural compound statins such as lovastatin, unsaturated fatty acids, sterols, and flavonoids. Xuezhikang Capsule has the effects of resolving turbidity and lowering lipid, promoting blood circulation to remove blood stasis, and invigorating the spleen and promoting digestion. It is especially suitable for patients with dyslipidemia with spleen deficiency, phlegm obstruction, and blood stasis manifested as shortness of breath, fatigue, dizziness, chest oppression, chest pain, abdominal distension, and poor appetite. China Coronary Secondary Prevention Study (CCSPS), led by Fuwai Hospital of the Chinese Academy of Medical Sciences, is a multicenter, randomized, double-blind, placebo-controlled clinical trial, involving a total of 4,870 coronary heart disease patients with a history of myocardial infarction. After an average of 3.5 years of treatment, it was found that Xuezhikang Capsule could reduce triglyceride by 13.2%, decrease low-density lipoprotein cholesterol by 20.2% and total cholesterol by 15.0%, and increase high-density lipoprotein cholesterol by 4.9%. Compared with placebo, Xuezhikang Capsule could reduce the risk of coronary heart disease events by 45%, coronary heart disease death by 31%, and all-cause death by 33%. The findings were published in the *Journal of the American College of Cardiology* in 2008. The medicine has been used clinically for over 20 years, and its efficacy and safety have been widely recognized. The administration method is to take 2 capsules orally each time, twice daily.

References

LU Z, KOU W, DU B, et al. Effect of Xuezhikang, an extract from red yeast Chinese rice, on coronary events in a Chinese population with previous myocardial infarction[J]. Am J Cardiol, 2008, 101 (12): 1689-1693.

4 Prediabetes mellitus

Pre-diabetes refers to the stage where impaired fasting glucose and abnormal glucose tolerance have appeared, but the diagnostic criteria for diabetes have not yet been reached. In China, more than one-third of people are in pre-diabetes. Without intervention, many patients will progress to diabetes, which will bring a heavy burden to the society.

In clinical manifestations, most do not have characteristic symptoms, and only abnormal fasting blood glucose, glucose tolerance test or glycosylated hemoglobin are found during physical examination.

In clinical diagnosis, people with impaired fasting glucose (FPG: 5.6–6.9 mmol/L) and impaired glucose tolerance (OGTT2hPG:7.8–11.0 mmol/L), or glycosylated hemoglobin 5.7%–6.4%, can be diagnosed as pre-diabetes.

Clinical treatment mainly includes lifestyle interventions such as balanced diet and doing exercise, and taking metformin to delay the progress of the disease. TCM believes that this abnormal metabolic disease has a lot to do with the constitution. TCM has certain curative effects and advantages in regulating constitution according to syndrome differentiation and actively treating pre-diabetes.

In TCM, pre-diabetes belongs to the category of "consumptive thirst". In etiology, it is related to the lack of congenital endowment, improper diet, fatigue, and internal injury. In pathogenesis, yin deficiency is the root cause, and dryness-heat is the manifestation.

In clinical treatment, Yuye Decoction, created by Zhang Xichun, a famous doctor in the Qing Dynasty, and Chinese patent medicine Tianqi Jiangtang Capsule are commonly used. Yuye Decoction is a famous prescription for decreasing blood glucose, which is composed of 7 Chinese medicinals: Huangqi (Astragali Radix), Tianhuafen (Trichosanthis Radix), Zhimu (Anemarrhenae Rhizoma), Gegen (Puerariae Lobatae Radix), Wuweizi (Schisandrae Chinensis Fructus), Shanyao (Dioscoreae Rhizoma) and Jineijn (Galli Gigerii Endothelium Corneum). This prescription has the effects of benefiting qi for promoting production of fluid, and strengthening the kidney and quenching thirst. It is suitable for pre-diabetic patients with deficiency of both qi and yin, manifested as thirst, excessive urination, fatigue, and feeble pulse. Modern pharmacological studies have found that Huangqi (Astragali Radix), Tianhuafen (Trichosanthis

Radix), Zhimu (Anemarrhenae Rhizoma), Gegen (Puerariae Lobatae Radix) and Wuweizi (Schisandrae Chinensis Fructus) in the prescription have a certain effect of decreasing blood glucose.

Tianqi Jiangtang Capsule is a Chinese patent medicine developed based on Yuye Decoction. It is composed of 10 Chinese medicinals, including Tianhuafen (Trichosanthis Radix), Huangqi (Astragali Radix), Nvzhenzi (Ligustri Lucidi Fructus), Shihu (Dendrobii Caulis), Renshen (Ginseng Radix et Rhizoma), Digupi (Lycii Cortex), Huanglian (Coptidis Rhizoma), Shanzhuyu (Corni Rructus), Mohanlian (Ecliptae Herba) and Wuweizi (Schisandrae Chinensis Fructus). It has the effects of benefiting qi and nourishing yin, and clearing heat and promoting production of fluid. This medcine is suitable for pre-diabetic patients with symptoms of deficiency of both qi and yin, such as burnout and fatigue, thirst, dysphoria with feverish sensation in the chest, palms and soles, spontaneous sweating, night sweating, palpitation, insomnia, reddish tongue, thin and dry fur, thready and weak or rapid pulse, etc. A randomized, double-blind, multicenter clinical study involving 420 pre-diabetic patients led by Academician Tong Xiaolin of Guang'anmen Hospital of China Academy of Chinese Medical Sciences showed that compared with placebo, taking Tianqi Jiangtang Capsule for 1 year could reduce the incidence of diabetes by 32.1%. The medicine is a hard capsule, and its contents are brown-yellow to brown powder and granules, with a slight fragrance and a bitter taste. The administration method is to take 5 capsules orally each time, 3 times daily.

References

LIAN F, LI G, CHEN X, et al. Chinese herbal medicine Tianqi reduces progression from impaired glucose tolerance to diabetes: a double-blind, randomized, placebo-controlled, multicenter trial[J]. J Clin Endocrinol Metab, 2014, 99 (2): 648-655.

5 Diabetes

Diabetes is a metabolic disease characterized by chronic hyperglycemia, which is caused by abnormal glucose metabolism due to insufficient insulin secretion or utilization defects under the influence of genetic and environmental factors. In the past ten years, the number of diabetes patients in China has increased from 90 million to 140 million. In 2021, the number of diabetes patients in the world was as high as 537 million, and the incidence rate showed a rapid upward trend in recent years, which has become a major global public health problem.

In clinical manifestations, diabetes can be divided into type 1 diabetes and type 2 diabetes. The former is more common in adolescence, with acute onset and apparent symptoms. The latter is generally after 40 years old, with insidious onset and mild symptoms. Whether type 1 or type 2, it can show typical "three more and one less", that is, drinking more, eating more, urinating more, and losing weight. In addition, diabetes is often accompanied by complications of various systems. Of course, there are also some patients who have no apparent symptoms and are only found by chance during a physical examination or medical visit.

In clinical diagnosis, the diagnosis of diabetes often takes "three more and one less", clinical manifestations of various common complications and family history of diabetes as clues, and diagnosis is made by fasting plasma glucose (FPG), random blood glucose, glycosylated hemoglobin (HbA1c), and oral glucose tolerance test (OGTT) 2-hour plasma glucose (2hPG) value.

In clinical treatment, besides lifestyle intervention, treating diabetes often includes insulin secretagogues, insulin sensitizers, α-glucosidase inhibitors, insulin, GLP-1 receptor agonists, and so on. TCM has certain curative effects and advantages in controlling hyperglycemia, improving metabolic disorder, and preventing related complications, so many patients will actively seek TCM treatment.

In TCM, diabetes belongs to the category of "consumptive thirst". In etiology, it is related to the insufficiency of congenital endowment, eating disorders, overstrain, and internal damage. In pathogenesis, yin deficiency is the root cause, dryness-heat are the manifestations, and yin deficiency involving yang and deficiency of both yin and yang may occur due to a long-term illness.

In clinical treatment, Gegen Qinlian Decoction and Chinese patent medicine Xiaoke Pill are often used. Gegen Qinlian Decoction comes from the medical book *Treatise on Cold Pathogenic Diseases* in the Han Dynasty, which is composed of 4 Chinese medicinals: Gegen (Puerariae Lobatae Radix), Huangqin (Scutellariae Radix), Huanglian (Coptidis Rhizoma) and Gancao (Glycyrrhizae Radix et Rhizoma). It has the effect of resolving superficies and clearing interior. This prescription was initially used to treat diarrhea caused by pathogenic qi penetrating inward due to non-recovery of cold. Modern clinical studies have found that Gegen Qinlian Decoction has an excellent hypoglycemic effect and is widely used to treat diabetes. This prescription is especially suitable for diabetic patients with the syndrome of dampness-heat in intestines based on TCM syndrome differentiation, accompanied by a bitter taste, polydipsia, diarrhea, red tongue with greasy yellow fur, slippery and rapid pulse, and other symptoms. A randomized, double-blind, controlled clinical trial involving 187 patients with type 2 diabetes was conducted by Academician Tong Xiaolin of Guang'anmen Hospital, China Academy of Chinese Medical Sciences. It was found that compared with the placebo group, Gegen Qinlian Decoction could significantly improve fasting blood glucose and glycosylated hemoglobin levels after 12 weeks of intervention and its mechanism of action was related to the regulation of intestinal microbiome.

Xiaoke Pill is a compound preparation of Chinese and Western medicines made by adding glyburide based on the traditional prescriptions of Yuquan Pill and Xiaoke Fang including 7 Chinese medicinals: Huangqi (Astragali Radix), Dihuang (Rehmanniae Radix), Shanyao (Dioscoreae Rhizoma), Gegen (Puerariae Lobatae Radix), Tianhuafen (Trichosanthis Radix), Yumixu (Stigma Maydis) and Wuweizi (Schisandrae Chinensis Fructus), which have the effects of nourishing kidney and yin and benefiting qi for promoting production of fluid. They can effectively reduce fasting blood glucose, 2-hour plasma glucose and glycosylated hemoglobin levels in diabetic patients. In addition, a randomized, controlled, double-blind, and multicenter clinical trial conducted by Professor Ji Linong of Peking University People's Hospital involved 800 patients with type 2 diabetes with poor blood sugar control. Compared with glyburide, Xiaoke Pill significantly reduced the risk of hypoglycemia and improved blood sugar level after 48 weeks of intervention, suggesting that the components in Xiaoke Pill have a protective effect on glyburide-induced hypoglycemia. Xiaoke Pill is suitable for diabetic patients with deficiency of both qi and yin according to TCM syndrome differentiation. Its clinical manifestations are spirit fatigue, fatigue, thirst, poor appetite, weakness, reddish tongue, thin and white fur, and feeble or thready and weak pulse. The specification is concentrated water pills, generally 120 per bottle and 2.5g per 10 pills. The dosage and administration method is 5–10 pills orally each time, 2–3 times daily.

References

XU J, LIAN F, ZHAO L, et al. Structural modulation of gut microbiota during alleviation of type 2 diabetes with a Chinese herbal formula[J]. ISME J, 2015, 9 (3): 552-562.

JI L, TONG X, WANG H, et al. Efficacy and safety of traditional Chinese medicine for diabetes: a double-blind, randomised, controlled trial[J]. PLoS One. 2013, 8 (2): e56703. doi: 10. 1371/journal. pone. 0056703.

6 Diabetic complications

In China, more than one-tenth people have diabetes, and 7 out of 10 people with diabetics have complications. Some people say that diabetes is not terrible, but diabetic complications are terrible, which is reasonable. Diabetes can cause chronic and progressive lesions in tissues and organs such as eyes, kidneys, blood vessels and nerves, leading to multi-system complications and even acute severe metabolic disorders.

In clinical manifestations, diabetes may cause acute and severe metabolic disorders, various chronic complications, and is more likely to be complicated with infectious diseases. Diabetic nephropathy and diabetic retinopathy may occur when microvessels are involved, and coronary heart disease, stroke, and renal arteriosclerosis may occur when cardio-cereal renal artery vessels are involved. Diabetic foot is a severe and scary complication with high treatment cost, often manifested as ulcer and gangrene that are difficult to heal for many patients, leading to their amputation.

In clinical treatment, according to different complications, choose the corresponding treatment scheme, including rehydration, correcting electrolyte disorder and acid-base imbalance, insulin, anti-infection, anti-heart failure, and so on. Especially, when dealing with diabetic foot, anti-infection, debridement and dressing change should be actively applied. TCM has a certain curative effect on improving diabetic complications. This paper introduces the understanding and treatment of TCM with the diabetic foot as an example.

In TCM, diabetic foot belongs to the category of "deteriorated case of consumptive thirst" and "gangrene of digit". In etiology and pathogenesis, diabetes lasts for a long time, causing damage to yin and yang, blood vessels stasis and stagnation, intermingled phlegm, blood stasis, and heat-toxin, which leads to decayed flesh, tendon and ligament exhaustion, and vanquished bone.

In clinical treatment, Simiao Yong'an Decoction is often used. This prescription comes from the Qing Dynasty medical book *New Compilation of Effective Recipes*, which is composed of Jinyinhua (Lonicerae Japonicae Flos), Xuanshen (Scrophulariae Radix), Danggui (Angelicae Sinensis Radix), and Gancao (Glycyrrhizae Radix et Rhizoma). It has the effects of clearing heat and removing toxicity, and promoting blood circulation to relieve pain. In the original book, it is mainly used for "gangrene of digit" with blazing heat-toxin. It is commonly used to treat lower limb diseases such as thromboangiitis obliterans, deep venous embolism of lower limbs, and diabetic foot. Modern

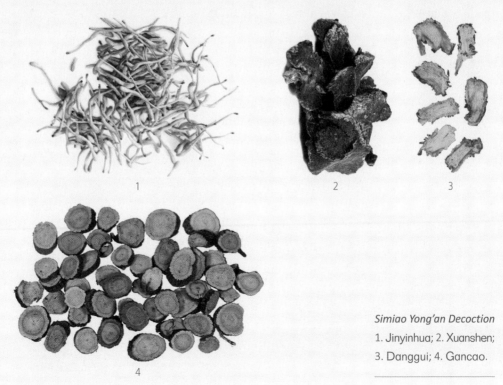

Simiao Yong'an Decoction
1. Jinyinhua; 2. Xuanshen;
3. Danggui; 4. Gancao.

pharmacological studies have found that Jinyinhua (Lonicerae Japonicae Flos), Xuanshen (Scrophulariae Radix), Danggui (Angelicae Sinensis Radix), and Gancao (Glycyrrhizae Radix et Rhizoma) have good anti-infection, anti-inflammatory and microcirculation improvement effects. It should be noted that although Simiao Yong'an Decoction has fewer medicinals, the dosage of each medicinal is large, which is the key to the effectiveness of this prescription. In practical use, combined with the basic pathogenesis of diabetic foot due to yin deficiency and dryness-heat, decayed flesh and vanquished blood, Chinese medicinals with the effects of nourishing yin, clearing heat, decreasing blood glucose, expressing toxin, expelling pus and promoting granulation can be added.

Section 7
Rheumatic Diseases

| Overview of rheumatic diseases

Rheumatic diseases are a group of diseases with different etiologies, but they all involve bones, joints, and their surrounding tissues. Its etiology is varied, including infection, immune disorders, endocrine disorders, environmental factors, genetic and degenerative diseases, and so on. Rheumatic diseases have a high incidence, a long course, a certain disability rate, and low mortality rate. In clinical symptoms, joint and soft tissue pain is one of the most common symptoms of rheumatic diseases, including joint stiffness, swelling, deformation, and limited movement.

Currently, medical therapy is the primary treatment means, often using non-steroidal anti-inflammatory medicines, glucocorticoids, and cytotoxic medicines. However, the disadvantage is excessive side effects, including gastrointestinal reactions, hepatotoxicity, infection, osteoporosis, bone marrow suppression, fetal teratogenicity, and so on. In recent years, although biologics have become one of the critical directions in treating rheumatic diseases as specific antagonists against pathogenic target molecules, they are expensive and difficult to be popularized on a large scale. Therefore, many patients with rheumatic immune system diseases will actively seek TCM treatment to relieve the symptom of limb joint pain. Even in the hospitals of Western medicine, Chinese patent medicines such as Leigongteng preparations are widely used.

In TCM, rheumatic diseases belong to the category of "bi syndrome". In etiology, TCM believes that this disease is caused by the deficiency of healthy qi first and then by the pathogenic wind, cold, dampness or other pathogens invading the joints and meridians. In pathogenesis, there is deficiency of vital qi and wind-cold-dampness pathogen, or stagnation transforming into heat, blocking meridians. In clinical treatment, strengthening vital qi to eliminate pathogenic factors is the primary treatment method. More and more clinical evidences show that TCM can improve clinical symptoms, reduce attack frequency and adverse reactions in treating rheumatic diseases, which has the clinical value that can not be ignored. This section will focus on TCM's understanding and treatment of rheumatoid arthritis, systemic lupus erythematosus, ankylosing spondylitis, Sjogren's syndrome, and Raynaud's disease.

‖ Treatises on rheumatic diseases

1 Rheumatoid arthritis

Rheumatoid arthritis, a systemic autoimmune disease, is characterized by symmetrical and persistent polyarthritis of small joints such as hands and wrists. Clinical manifestations are stiffness, pain and swelling of joints in the morning. If not actively treated, joint deformity and loss of function can be caused. It can often involve organs and tissues such as heart, lung, kidney and nervous system, and various nervous system manifestations caused by rheumatoid nodules and vasculitis, pulmonary interstitial lesions, pericarditis, myocarditis, and compression of rheumatoid nodules can appear. In China, the incidence ranges from 0.2%–0.4%, and can be seen at any age, especially from 30–50 years old, and the ratio of females to males is about 3：1.

In etiology, infection and autoimmune reaction are the central links to this disease, and genetic, endocrine, and environmental factors can increase its susceptibility. The primary pathogenesis is an immune disorder.

In clinical treatment, commonly used medicines include non-steroidal anti-inflammatory medicines, antirheumatic medicines, immunosuppressants, glucocorticoids, and biologics. Methotrexate is a widely used medicine at present. However, many patients are intolerant to its accompanying gastrointestinal reactions, hepatorenal toxicity, infection, osteoporosis, bone marrow suppression, and other discomforts.

In TCM, this disease belongs to the category of "pain of multiple joints" and "Wangbi". In etiology and pathogenesis, vital qi is deficient first, and then pathogenic qi such as wind, cold, dampness, and heat blocks meridians.

In clinical treatment, Chinese patent medicine Leigongteng polyglycosides, as well as classic prescriptions Mahuang Jiazhu Decoction and Duhuo Jisheng Decoction are commonly used.

Leigongteng polyglycosides, known as "Chinese herbal medicine hormone", is the first Chinese medicinal preparation with anti-inflammatory and immunomodulatory effects extracted from the xylem of the root of Celastraceae plant *Tripterygium wilfordii* Hook. F. in China, which is also a fat-soluble mixture. Its physiological activity is produced by the synergistic superposition of diterpene lactones, alkaloids, triterpenes, and other active components, which not only has an immunosuppressive effect, but also removes toxic components. It has been widely used in treating rheumatoid arthritis, primary glomerulonephropathy, nephrotic syndrome, lupus nephritis, lupus erythematosus, subacute and chronic severe hepatitis, chronic active hepatitis, and other diseases. In 2012, Peking Union Medical College Hospital carried out a randomized, controlled, and clinical study on treating active rheumatoid arthritis with Leigongteng polyglycosides, which included 207 patients. It was found that after 24 weeks of treatment, the effective treatment rate of the Leigongteng group alone was 55.1%, which was higher than that of the methotrexate group alone (46.4%), while the effective treatment rate of the methotrexate combined with Leigongteng was as high as 76.8 %. Studies have confirmed that for active rheumatoid arthritis, the curative effect of Leigongteng polyglycosides alone is no less than that of methotrexate alone, and the curative effect of combined use of Leigongteng polyglycosides and methotrexate is significantly better than that of methotrexate alone. There is no significant difference in the incidence of adverse reactions among different medicine groups. The only thing worth noting is that taking Leigongteng for a long time has certain toxicity to gonads, so unmarried and childless people should use it cautiously. The clinical dosage is 0.3–0.5 mg/kg per time, usually 1–2 tablets, 3 times daily after meals.

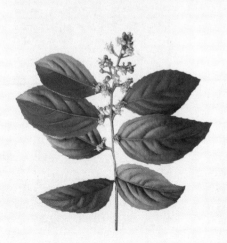

Mahuang Jiazhu Decoction, a famous classic prescription, comes from *Synopsis of Golden Chamber*, which is composed of Mahuang (Ephedrae Herba), Guizhi (Cinnamomi Ramulus), Xingren (Armeniacae Semen Amarum), Baizhu (Atractylodis

Source plant of Leigongteng

Macrocephalae Rhizoma) and Gancao (Glycyrrhizae Radix et Rhizoma). It has the effects of dispelling cold and removing dampness, and invigorating the spleen and warming yang. This prescription can be used for treating wind-cold-dampness bi syndrome of rheumatoid arthritis when the clinical manifestations of patients are pain and swelling of joints, fever, loss of appetite, white and greasy fur, and floating and tight pulse. The exterior syndrome is apparent, which is similar to the cold. When manifestations are aggravated due to cold pathogen, this prescription can be considered.

Duhuo Jisheng Decoction comes from *Essential Recipes for Emergent Use Worth A Thousand Gold*, which is composed of Duhuo (Angelicae Pubescentis Radix), Sangjisheng (Taxilli Herba), Qinjiao (Gentianae Macrophyllae Radix), Fangfeng (Saposhnikoviae Radix), Xixin (Asari Radix et Rhizoma), Chuanxiong (Chuanxiong Rhizoma), Danggui (Angelicae Sinensis Radix), Shengdihuang (Rehmanniae Radix), Baishao (Paeoniae Radix Alba), Rougui (Cinnamomi Cortex), Fuling (Poria), Duzhong (Eucommiae Cortex), Niuxi (Achyranthis Bidentatae Radix), Renshen (Ginseng Radix et Rhizoma) and Gancao (Glycyrrhizae Radix et Rhizoma). This prescription has the functions of dispelling wind-dampness, relieving painful bi, tonifying the liver and kidney and invigorating qi and blood. In treating rheumatoid arthritis, if accompanied by limb joint soreness, aggravation due to cold pathogen, waist and knee pain, soreness and weakness, unfavorable flexion and extension of limbs, aversion to cold and affection for warmth, palpitation, and shortness of breath, this prescription can be considered.

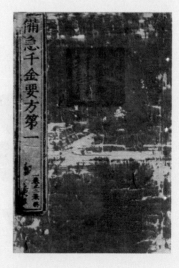

Essential Recipes for Emergent Use Worth A Thousand Gold
(Bèi Jí Qiān Jīn Yào Fāng, 备急千金要方)
Preserved in China Academy of Chinese Medical Sciences (CACMS)

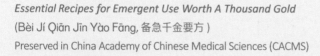

References

LYU Q W, ZHANG W, SHI Q, et al. Comparison of Tripterygium wilfordii Hook F with methotrexate in the treatment of active rheumatoid arthritis (TRIFRA): a randomised, controlled clinical trial[J]. Annals of the Rheumatic Diseases, 2015, 74(6): 1-9.

2 Systemic lupus erythematosus

Systemic lupus erythematosus is an autoimmune disease, characterized by immune inflammation and diffuse connective tissue disease, which can cause damage to many organs and tissues of the human body. In China, the prevalence rate is (30.13 –70.41) / 100,000, which is more common in women of childbearing age, and pregnancy can also induce this disease.

Its pathogenesis is still unclear, possibly related to genetic, endocrine, and environmental factors. Environmental factors can be seen in chemicals, virus infection, and so on.

In clinical symptoms, the primary manifestations include facial characteristic butterfly erythema, common oral or nasal mucosal ulcer, long-term low to moderate fever, symmetrical multi-joint pain and swelling, but generally will not cause bone damage, and migraine. In severe cases, cerebrovascular accidents, epilepsy, coma, etc., can appear. In addition, it also includes inflammation of various tissues and organs of the whole body, such as lupus nephritis, lupus pneumonia, pericarditis, enteritis, acute pancreatitis, and conjunctivitis. This disease can lead to death from multiple organ failure and infection in the acute stage.

Clinical treatment includes non-steroidal anti-inflammatory medicines, antimalarial medicines, hormones, immunosuppressants, new drug biologics, immunoglobulins, plasma exchange, hematopoietic stem cell transplantation, and so on. However, clinical findings showed that some patients were intolerant to the adverse reactions caused by the above treatment, including digestive tract ulcers, bleeding, liver and kidney injuries, fundus lesions, rashes, and so on.

In the outpatient service, patients mainly seek TCM treatment to improve clinical symptoms, and reduce complications and side effects.

In TCM, systemic lupus erythematosus belongs to the categories of "yin-yang toxics", "warm-toxin disease with ecchymoses", and "lupus erythematosus and flowing turbidity". In etiology, it is related to the invasion of external toxin, congenital deficiency, the combination of the external and internal pathogen, and long-term retention of toxin and pathogen in the body to damage zang-fu viscera. In pathogenesis, deficiency of true yin is the root cause, and blood stasis, toxin, and phlegm obstruction are the manifestations.

Clinically, the classic prescription Xijiao Dihuang Decoction and Chinese patent medicine Baishao Glycosides Capsule are commonly used. Xijiao Dihuang Decoction comes from *Arcane Essentials from the Imperial Library*, which is composed of Xijiao (Cornu Rhinocerotis) (now replaced by Shui niu jiao; Cornu Bubali), Dihuang (Rehmanniae Radix), Baishao (Paeoniae Radix Alba) and Mudanpi (Moutan Cortex). It has the effects of clearing heat and removing toxicity, and cooling blood and dissipating blood stasis. Modern pharmacological research shows that this prescription has sedative, anticonvulsant, and analgesic effects, and can prevent epilepsy, coma, and other symptoms caused by systemic lupus erythematosus. The prescription has a protective effect on the cardiovascular system, nervous system, and other multi-system organs, and also has critical auxiliary effects such as anti-inflammation, hemostasis and improving normal immunity and systemic organ damage caused by lupus. The paeonia glycosides in Baishao (Paeoniae Radix Alba) have anti-inflammatory and bidirectional immunomodulatory effects, and are also the primary components for treating this disease; when lupus erythematosus patients have butterfly erythema, joint pain, body heat, delirium, dysphoria, and other symptoms, this prescription can be considered.

Paeonia Glycosides Capsule is a mixture of glycosides with physiological functions extracted from Baishao (Paeoniae Radix Alba). Because of its bidirectional regulation of the immune system, it is widely used as auxiliary medicine for autoimmune diseases such as rheumatoid arthritis, systemic lupus erythematosus, and ankylosing spondylitis. A clinical treatment study of paeonia glycosides in the lupus active stage, which included 978 lupus patients, showed that the medicine could significantly improve lupus activity score within 1–6 months, and then steadily maintain and improve symptoms. Moreover, it can also reduce 24-hour urinary protein, which has a certain renal protection effect. The medicine is a natural extract, and no related adverse reactions have been observed, so it can be taken for a long time. Very few patients may have digestive symptoms, but most can relieve themselves. This medicine is used orally, 2 capsules at a time, 2–3 times daily.

References

CHEN Y F, WANG L D, CAO Y, et al. Paeonia lactiflora total glucosides of for safely reducing disease activity in systemic lupus erythematosus: a systematic review and meta-analysis[J]. Front Pharmacol, 2022, 13: e834947. doi: 10. 3389/fphar. 2022. 834947.

3 Ankylosing spondylitis

Ankylosing spondylitis is chronic inflammatory rheumatism with axial spinal joint involvement in spinal arthritis, possibly accompanied by extra-articular manifestations, and severe cases may have spinal ankylosis and deformity. In etiology, the disease is a polygenic genetic disease caused by genetic and environmental factors. This disease has a strong familial aggregation. Environmental factors are mainly related to inflammation and the immune response caused by intestinal pathogens such as chlamydia and salmonella. In China, the prevalence rate is about 0.25%. The ratio of males to females is 1 : 1, and the males are more seriously ill.

Pathologically, this disease is characterized by repeated inflammation, fibrosis, and even ossification of tendons, ligaments, and joint capsules in various bone and joint parts, and is more common in the heel, palm, knee joint, chest rib, spine, iliac crest, greater trochanter of femur, ischial tubercle, and so on.

In clinical symptoms, the early manifestation is low back pain with morning stiffness, or radioactive soreness from buttocks and groin to lower limbs, which is relieved after activity. With the progression of the disease, there may be limited movement in all directions of the lumbar and thoracic spine. Extra-articular symptoms include iritis and aortic valve disease, and in a few patients renal dysfunction, pneumonia, and muscle atrophy can be found.

In clinical treatment, this disease generally does not affect life span, but the disability rate is high. The disease responds well to non-steroidal anti-inflammatory medicines, which is the first-line medicine in the clinic. However, the course of this disease is long, and the side effects brought by long-term use of such drugs often make patients unbearable, so some patients come for TCM treatment.

In TCM, ankylosing spondylitis belongs to the category of "kyphosis" and "bi syndrome". In etiology, it is related to congenital deficiency and externally contracted dampness toxin. In pathogenesis, kidney deficiency and stagnant blockade of dampness-heat are the primary factors.

In treatment, the classic prescriptions Jingui Shenqi Pill and Guizhi Shaoyao Zhimu Decoction are commonly used to treat both manifestation and root cause.

Jingui Shenqi Pill comes from *Synopsis of Golden Chamber*, which is composed of Dihuang (Rehmanniae Radix), Shanzhuyu (Corni Rructus), Shanyao (Dioscoreae Rhizoma), Mudanpi (Moutan Cortex), Zexie (Alismatis Rhizoma), Fuling (Poria), Guizhi (Cinnamomi Ramulus) and Zhifuzi (dried Aconiti Lateralis Radix Praeparata). It has the functions of invigorating the kidney and reinforcing yang, and warming qi to move water. Clinically, it can be used for patients with ankylosing spondylitis accompanied by soreness and weakness of the waist and knees, fear of cold and cold limbs, joint pain, edema of lower limbs, and dysuria. Pharmacological studies have found that Jingui Shenqi Pill can regulate immune response. This prescription is often used in the remission stage of ankylosing spondylitis. Now, this prescription has been developed into the form of Chinese patent medicine water-honeyed pills. The dosage and administration method is to take 20 capsules (4g)–25 capsules (5g) orally each time and twice daily.

Guizhi Shaoyao Zhimu Decoction also comes from *Synopsis of Golden Chamber*, which is composed of Guizhi (Cinnamomi Ramulus), Shaoyao (Paeoniae Radix Alba seu Rubra), Zhimu (Anemarrhenae Rhizoma), Gancao (Glycyrrhizae Radix et Rhizoma), Mahuang (Ephedrae Herba), Shengjiang (Zingiberis Rhizoma Recens), Baizhu (Atractylodis Macrocephalae Rhizoma), Zhifuzi (dried Aconiti Lateralis Radix Praeparata) and Fangfeng (Saposhnikoviae Radix). It has the effects of dispelling wind and removing dampness, and dispelling cold and unblocking yang. Modern pharmacological studies have shown that Guizhi Shaoyao Zhimu

Decoction can improve symptoms from analgesia, anti-inflammation, immune regulation, and has the effects of protecting bones and joints and relieving bone and joint injury. Clinically, it can be used to treat patients with ankylosing spondylitis in remission stage with limb pain, joint enlargement, emaciation, nausea and vomiting, dizziness, limited movement of spine and thorax, reddish tongue, thin and white fur, and stringy and thready pulse. It also has a good effect on the prevention and treatment of ankylosing spondylitis in the acute attack period. Clinical manifestations such as "redness, swelling, heat and pain" of joints, dysfunction of activities, abnormal renal function caused by inflammation and elevated blood uric acid can be seen. Studies have found that Guizhi Shaoyao Zhimu Decoction can protect renal function, accelerate uric acid excretion, resist inflammation and relieve pain.

4 Sjogren's syndrome

Sjogren's syndrome is a chronic inflammatory autoimmune disease that invades exocrine glands such as lacrimal and salivary glands. In China, the prevalence rate of Sjogren's syndrome is 0.29%–0.77%, which can occur at any age, and is more common in 30–60 years old.

Currently, the etiology and pathogenesis are unclear, but genetic, infectious, and environmental factors are all involved in its pathogenesis. The primary pathological reactions are autoimmune reactions and inflammation-mediated tissue damage, especially in exocrine glands. Generally, the prognosis limited to exocrine glands is better, and visceral injury can endanger life if not treated timely.

Clinical manifestations, including keratitis xerosis and xerostomia, can involve internal organs, and there are also systemic manifestations, including rash, joint pain, renal calcification, kidney stones and other kidney diseases, xero-pharyngitis, atrophic gastritis, motor nerve abnormality, hemiplegia, hemocytopenia, thyroiditis, pneumonia, and other multi-system involvement symptoms.

In clinical treatment, there is no cure at present. Replacement therapy of glandular secretions such as artificial tears, artificial saliva, gel and others are applied to relieve symptoms; immunosuppressants are used to control systemic autoimmune reaction symptoms, glucocorticoids in severe cases; non-steroidal anti-inflammatory medicines are commonly used to treat muscle and joint pain as well as other symptomatic treatments. However, we have found that many patients are intolerant to the side effects because of the lifelong use of medication. In order to improve clinical symptoms and quality of life and reduce side effects, they often actively seek TCM treatment.

In TCM, Sjogren's syndrome belongs to the categories of "dryness syndrome", "dryness bi" and "dryness toxin". In etiology, it is related to congenital endowment deficiency, emotions transforming into fire, exogenous dryness pathogen, yin deficiency of liver and kidney, etc. In pathogenesis, yin deficiency of the liver and kidney, deficiency of qi and fluid, and blockade of blood stasis are related.

In treatment, classic prescriptions such as Yiguanjian Decoction and Qiju Dihuang Pill are commonly used in the clinic. In addition, if the systemic symptoms are apparent, it is of great significance to use Leigongteng Polyglycosides Tablet or Paeonia Glycosides Capsule to relieve symptoms and prevent disease development.

Yiguanjian Decoction comes from the *Supplement to Classified Case Records of Celebrated Physicians* written by Wei Zhixiu, a famous doctor in the Qing Dynasty. This prescription is composed of Dihuang (Rehmanniae Radix), Beishashen (Glehniae Radix), Maidong (Ophiopogonis Radix), Danggui (Angelicae Sinensis Radix), Gouqizi (Lycii Fructus) and Chuanlianzi (Toosendan Fructus). It has the effects of nourishing yin and dispersing stagnated liver qi. Clinically, it is mainly used for Sjogren's syndrome with yin deficiency of the liver and kidney and constraint and stagnation of liver qi, characterized by dry mouth and throat, red tongue and little fluid, and chest and hypochondriac pain. Modern pharmacological studies have shown that Yiguanjian Decoction can alleviate gland injury and repair gland secretion function.

Qiju Dihuang Pill is made by adding Gouqizi (Lycii Fructus) and Juhua (Chrysanthemi Flos) based on Liuwei Dihuang Pill, including Gouqizi (Lycii Fructus), Juhua (Chrysanthemi Flos), Shudihuang (Rehmanniae Radix Praeparata), wine-prepared Shanzhuyu (Corni Rructus), Mudanpi (Moutan Cortex), Shanyao (Dioscoreae Rhizoma), Fuling (Poria) and Zexie (Alismatis Rhizoma). This prescription can nourish the kidney and liver, and is used for Sjogren's syndrome with yin deficiency of the liver and kidney. Its clinical manifestations are photophobia, red and dry eyes, dim vision, dizziness, tinnitus, etc. Modern pharmacological studies have shown that Qiju Dihuang Pill has a better protective effect on the kidney, and has a certain effect on preventing severe kidney damage induced by Sjogren's syndrome. Qiju Dihuang Pill is generally concentrated pills. Each 8 pills is equivalent to 3 g of the raw medicinal materials, and each bottle has 200 pills with oral administration of 8 pills each time and three times a day.

5 Raynaud's disease

Raynaud's disease is a spasmodic disease of the small arterioles of the extremities caused by vascular and neurological dysfunction, which is not accompanied by systemic manifestations and is mainly primary. Secondary diseases often appear as symptoms of various immune diseases or connective tissue diseases, nervous system diseases, and chronic occlusive artery diseases, known as Raynaud's phenomenon. This disease is more common in women, the ratio of males to females is 1 : 10, and the age of onset is 20–30 years old.

Under the influence of cold or mental stimulation the skin at the distal end of limbs, e.g., the palm appears symmetrical, paroxysmal pallor, cyanotic changes, numbness, and tingling, and flushes after keeping warm.

In etiology, the pathogenesis of Raynaud's disease is still unclear. Currently, it is believed mainly related to genetic, immune and environmental factors. Cold and emotional stimulation are critical inducing factors, and other inducing factors are infection and fatigue. Early Raynaud's disease does not cause severe consequences.

Clinical treatment includes the local external use of 2% nitroglycerin ointment and compound heparin gel. Systematic medicines include vascular smooth muscle relaxants, peripheral vasodilators, 5-hydroxytryptamine antagonists, etc. If gangrene occurs, amputation may be required. The autoimmune reaction often leads to a long disease course and poor prognosis. Moreover, because of the disorder of vegetative nervous function, many patients show insomnia, dreaminess, irritability, and depression. These patients are mainly treated with TCM based on Western medicine control, which can improve various symptoms caused by neurological dysfunction and reduce side effects.

In TCM, Raynaud's disease belongs to the categories of "pulse bi", "blood bi" and "syncope". In etiology, it is related to congenital endowment deficiency, having a cold due to yang deficiency, emotional disorder, and other factors. In pathogenesis, it is related to yang deficiency of the spleen and kidney, deficiency of qi and blood, blockade of cold pathogen, and unsmooth blood circulation.

In clinical treatment, the classic prescriptions Yanghe Decoction and Huangqi Guizhi Wuwu Decoction are commonly used. Yanghe Decoction comes from the *Life-Saving Manual of Diagnosis and Treatment of External Diseases*, which is composed of Shudihuang (Rehmanniae Radix Praeparata), Lujiaojiao (Cervi Cornus Colla), Jiangtan (charred Zingiberis Rhizoma), Rougui (Cinnamomi Cortex), Mahuang (Ephedrae Herba), Baijiezi (Sinapis Semen) and Shenggancao (Glycyrrhizae Radix et Rhizoma). This prescription has the effects of warming yang, enriching blood, and dispelling cold and unblocking stagnation. It can be used for Raynaud's disease with cyanosis or pallor, aggravation due to cold pathogen, numbness and pain, lack of thirst in mouth, pale tongue with white fur, and deep and thready pulse. Especially when there is a gangrene tendency, it can be used. Modern pharmacological studies have shown that Yanghe Decoction can reduce the level of inflammatory factors and oxidative stress, alleviate neuropathic inflammation and has a good curative effect on peripheral neurodegenerative diseases and immune system diseases.

Huangqi Guizhi Wuwu Decoction comes from *Synopsis of Golden Chamber*, which is composed of Huangqi (Astragali Radix), Guizhi (Cinnamomi Ramulus), Shaoyao (Paeoniae Radix Alba seu Rubra), Shengjiang (Zingiberis Rhizoma Recens) and Dazao (Jujubae Fructus). It has the functions of warming channels for removing obstruction in collaterals, promoting blood circulation for relieving pain, and invigorating qi for consolidating wei qi. Modern pharmacological studies have also shown that this prescription has anti-inflammatory, analgesic, and vascular endothelium protection, immunity enhancement effects. It has a good curative effect on peripheral neuropathy. This prescription can be used for Raynaud's disease accompanied by fatigue, sweating, palpitation and dysphoria, dizziness, tinnitus, numbness or pain in extremities, dark red tongue, feeble or stringy pulse, etc.

Section 8
Nervous System Diseases

I Overview of nervous system diseases

Many people have had sudden hand numbness, leg numbness and limb shaking, possibly related to nervous system diseases. The so-called nervous system diseases include diseases occurring in the central nervous system, peripheral nervous system and autonomic nervous system, and can also be manifested as consciousness disorder, sensory disorder, motor disorder, abnormal muscle tone, etc. Among them, motor disorders can be manifested as paralysis and involuntary movement.

Nervous system diseases have a wide range of lesions, referring to the nerve parts of the whole body. Common clinical neurological diseases include cerebral infarction, transient ischemic attack, cerebral hemorrhage, amyotrophic lateral sclerosis, Parkinson's syndrome, epilepsy, progressive muscular dystrophy, ataxia, and so on. It is worth noting that nervous system diseases are very complex, and are difficult to diagnose or treat clinically. Moreover, due to the high mortality and disability rate caused by nervous system diseases, the functional recovery of patients has become a clinically recognized medical problem.

TCM has a unique cognitive system for the etiology and pathogenesis of nervous system diseases. According to TCM, this is closely related to wind pathogen, including internal wind and external wind. This is specially discussed in *The Yellow Emperor's Inner Classic*, including "pathogenic wind", "sudden stroke" and "hemiplegia". It is also pointed out in the *Synopsis of the Golden Chamber*, "the disease caused by wind pathogen is manifested by hemiplegia or inflexible arm movements, which is bi. Faint and rapid pulse is caused by stroke." In treatment, TCM also has a certain curative effect in promoting the recovery of the patients' limb function and improving their quality of life. This section will discuss the TCM recognition and treatment scheme of cerebral infarction and dizziness.

‖ Treatises on nervous system diseases

1 Cerebral infarction

Cerebral infarction, also known as ischemic stroke, refers to cerebrovascular disease with cerebral artery blood flow interruption, local brain tissue hypoxia and ischemic necrosis due to various reasons, which leads to corresponding neurological deficit. Cerebral infarction accounts for about 80% of all strokes. Common causes of cerebral infarction include atherosclerosis, cardiogenic embolism, arteriolar occlusion, and so on. Clinically, the common types of cerebral infarction include cerebral thrombosis, lacunar infarction, and cerebral embolism. The disease not only poses a great threat to human health, but also brings a heavy burden to patients and society.

In clinical symptoms, this disease is more common in middle-aged and elderly people aged 45–70. Acute onset often occurs, and the severity of symptoms is related to the location of brain damage, the size of cerebral ischemic blood vessels and the severity of ischemia. Mild cases may have no symptoms, while severe cases may show neurological dysfunction, including sudden fainting, unconsciousness, hemiplegia, speech disorder, mental retardation, hemianopia, dizziness, facial paralysis, ataxia, incontinence, and so on.

In clinical diagnosis, it is necessary to combine the patient's previous medical history, clinical manifestations, brain CT, MRI, transcranial Doppler ultrasound, carotid color B-ultrasound, magnetic resonance, angiography, digital subtraction cerebral angiography, carotid angiography, etc., to clarify a diagnosis.

Clinical treatment includes thrombolysis in the acute stage, intravascular intervention, antithrombosis, anticoagulation, dilatation, and standardized secondary preventive medical treatment. The prognosis of cerebral infarction is different, and the prognosis of small vessel occlusion is generally better.

It is worth noting that this disease has a high disability rate and high mortality rate, and its thrombolytic therapy has a strict time window. Many patients have missed the best time for thrombolysis when they seek medical treatment. In addition, some patients are intolerant to aspirin and statins, and the adverse reactions of Western medicines limit their clinical application to a certain extent.

In the acute stage and recovery stage of cerebral infarction, early intervention of TCM, including acupuncture and moxibustion can improve limb function, promote recovery, improve quality of life and reduce mortality to a certain extent.

Cerebral infarction belongs to the category of "apoplexy" in TCM. In etiology, it is mainly caused by reversed flow and disorder of qi and blood due to deficiency of vital qi, eating disorders, emotional disorder, overstrain, and internal damage, which leads to endogenous pathological factors such as wind, fire, phlegm, and blood stasis, blocking meridians. According to the degree of mental impairment, this disease can be divided into apoplexy involving channel and collateral and apoplexy involving zang-fu viscera.

In the clinic, the classic prescription Angong Niuhuang Pill can be used early in the acute stage, and acupuncture, massage, and other treatment measures can be combined in the convalescence stage. Angong Niuhuang Pill comes from *Systematic Differentiation of Warm Diseases* written by Wu Jutong, a doctor in the Qing Dynasty. It is one of the famous "three treasures of cold formula resuscitation" in TCM and an excellent first aid medicine for acute cerebral infarction. The medicine is composed of Niuhuang (Bovis Calculus), concentrated powder of Shuiniujiao (Bubali Cornu), artificial Shexiang (Moschus), Zhenzhu (Margarita), Zhusha (Cinnabaris), Xionghuang (Realgar), Huanglian (Coptidis Rhizoma), Huangqin (Scutellariae Radix), Zhizi (Gardeniae Fructus), Yujin (Curcumae Radix) and Bingpian (Borneolum Syntheticum), which can clear heat and remove toxicity, and suppress fright for resuscitation. In the acute stage of cerebral infarction, if there is high fever and dysphoria, unconsciousness and delirium, trismus, hemiplegia, red face and eyes, gruff breathing, wheezing due to retention of phlegm in the throat, red tongue and slippery pulse, which is the typical syndrome of "invasion of pericardium by heat", this prescription can be considered.

Acupuncture, massage and other TCM physiotherapy methods have unique curative effects on sequelae such as inflexible limb movements, inarticulateness, insomnia, numbness and pain, muscle spasm or weakness caused by cerebral infarction. In the selection of acupoints based on syndrome differentiation, the head acupoints are often Bǎihuì (GV20), Sìshéncōng (EX-HN1), Shéntíng (GV24), Yìntáng (GV29), Tàiyáng (EX-HN2) and Fēngchí (GB20); combined with inarticulateness or dysphagia, Chéngjiāng (CV24) and Liánquán (CV23) are often selected; combined with central facial paralysis, Dìcāng (ST4) and Jiáchē (ST6) are often selected. On the acupoints of limbs, Qūchí (LI11), Shǒusānlǐ (LI10), Wàiguān (TE5), Nèiguān (PC6), Shénmén (HT7), Hégǔ (LI4) and Hòuxī (SI3) can be taken from the upper limbs; Xuèhǎi (SP10), Liángqiū (ST34), Yīnlíngquán (SP9), Yánglíngquán (GB34), Zúsānlǐ (ST36), Shàngjùxū (ST37), Xiàjùxū (ST39), Sānyīnjiāo (SP6), Jiěxī (ST41), Zhàohǎi (KI6), Kūnlún (BL60), Tàichōng (LR3), Tàibái (SP3) can be taken from the lower limbs.

References

XIONG X J. Conotation of ancient "stroke" and Experience from *Qianyin Yaofang* Xiaoxuming Decoction treating cerebral infarction and cerebral hemorrhage[J]. Chinese Journal of TCM, 2020, 45 (12): 2735-2751.

2 Dizziness

In the outpatient clinic, many people suddenly realize that they can't control themselves or even stand due to dizziness, wondering if they are having cerebral infarction or is there anything wrong with them? This is especially common in the elderly people. After coming to the outpatient clinic for examination, they are often considered to be with mixed causes, including cerebral infarction, cerebral artery insufficiency, cervical spondylosis, and other diseases. Clinically, what is dizziness? What diseases are included?

Dizziness is a common clinical symptom, which can be manifested as dizziness, head distension, lightheadedness, and accompanied by fatigue, insomnia, tinnitus, forgetfulness, and other discomforts. The causes of dizziness are more complex, including cerebral ischemia, brain trauma, cerebral arteriosclerosis, vertebrobasilar insufficiency, neurasthenia, hypertension, hypotension, cervical spondylosis, hypoglycemia, epilepsy, anemia, infection, poisoning, Meniere's disease, arrhythmia, heart failure, autonomic nerve dysfunction, medicine poisoning, and so on.

In clinical diagnosis, for patients with dizziness, based on a detailed understanding of medical history and comprehensive physical examination, vestibular function, fundus, electrocardiogram, EEG, and CT examinations of head and cervical spine can be performed to investigate the cause.

In TCM, dizziness belongs to the categories of "intermittent headache" and "vertigo", which is closely related to emotional internal damage, eating disorders, head trauma or surgery, physical weakness, long-term illness, blood loss, overstrain, and so on. In pathogenesis, it is related to the deficiency of qi and blood and kidney essence, which leads to the emptiness of brain marrow and malnutrition of clear orifices, or upper hyperactivity of liver yang, the adverse rising of phlegm-fire and static blood blocking orifices, causing the disturbance of clear orifices.

In clinical treatment, the classic prescriptions Zexie Decoction and Guipi Decoction are commonly used. Zexie Decoction comes from the *Synopsis of Golden Chamber* written by Zhang Zhongjing. This prescription is composed of Zexie (Alismatis Rhizoma) and Baizhu (Atractylodis Macrocephalae Rhizoma). It has the effects of promoting urination to remove fluid retention and invigorating the spleen to control water. In ancient times, this prescription was used to treat "if a person has thoracic fluid retention in the epigastrium below the heart, it means he suffers from dizziness". That is to say, if patients present with vertigo, many cases of which are caused by fluid, then this prescription can be considered. We now use it to treat various types of dizziness, such as cerebral infarction, hypertension, cervical spondylosis and cerebral blood supply insufficiency, which can significantly improve dizziness symptoms. Zexie Decoction was once used to treat a patient with cervical spondylosis complicated with cerebral blood supply insufficiency, who was dizzy and could not walk. After taking this decoction, he did not faint on the same day. There are many similar experiences.

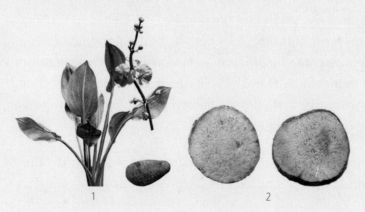

Zexie
1. Source plant;
2. decoction pieces.

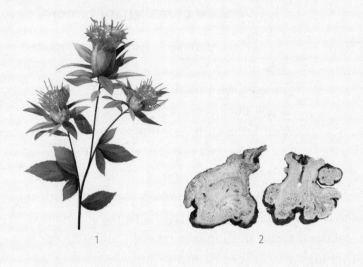

Baizhu
1. Source plant;
2. decoction pieces.

Guipi Decoction is also a classic prescription, which comes from the *Categorized Synopsis of the Whole*. Guipi Decoction is composed of Baizhu (Atractylodis Macrocephalae Rhizoma), Renshen (Ginseng Radix et Rhizoma), Huangqi (Astragali Radix), Danggui (Angelicae Sinensis Radix), Gancao (Glycyrrhizae Radix et Rhizoma), Fuling (Poria), Yuanzhi (Polygalae Radix), Suanzaoren (Ziziphi Spinosae Semen), Muxiang (Aucklandiae Radix), Longyanrou (Longan Arillus), Shengjiang (Zingiberis Rhizoma Recens), and Dazao (Jujubae Fructus), which has the effects of invigorating qi and enriching blood, and invigorating the spleen and nourishing the heart. For dizziness patients manifested by palpitation, insomnia, forgetfulness, night sweating, burnout and fatigue, poor appetite, sallow complexion without luster, pale tongue, thin and white fur, and thready and weak pulse, this prescription can be considered. We have found that patients with low blood pressure and weak constitution are often treated with this prescription. Chinese patent medicine Guipi Pill comes from this prescription— Guipi Decoction The commonly used method is oral administration. Take it with warm boiled water or ginger soup. 6 g of water-honeyed pills, 9 g of the small honey pills, and 1 large honey pill each time, 3 times daily.

Of course, there are many types of dizziness including hypertension-induced dizziness. In the treatment, we will choose the corresponding Chinese medicinals that can improve dizziness and reduce blood pressure; for patients with autonomic nerve dysfunction, anxiety, and depression, it is also necessary to choose the corresponding Chinese medicinals according to their anxiety state.

Section 9
Malignant Tumors

I Overview of malignant tumors

Malignant tumor is also known as cancer. When it comes to cancer, many people turn pale at the mention of cancer, and even many doctors think it is a "medical failure" and an insurmountable medical problem. According to the statistics of the World Health Organization in 2019, cancer is the first or second leading cause of death in most countries in the world, which brings a heavy disease burden to all countries. According to the latest statistical report of China's National Cancer Center in 2022, there were 4.064 million new cancer cases in China in 2016, with a world standard incidence rate of 186.46 / 100,000. The incidence rate of men was significantly higher than that of women. In 2016, the total number of cancer deaths was 2.414 million, and the world standard mortality rate was 105.19 / 100,000. The mortality rate of men was almost twice as high as that of women. Lung cancer, liver cancer, and gastric cancer are the top three causes of death, accounting for more than 40% of all cancer deaths.

Cancer in the early stage is not accompanied by apparent symptoms, such as early lung cancer, liver cancer, and gastric cancer, which is often found accidentally by CT, endoscopy and other examinations. As the disease progresses, when the tumor enlarges or invades other tissues and organs, it may appear symptoms such as apparent emaciation, bloody phlegm, progressive dysphagia, jaundice, and pain. In clinical treatment, chemotherapy, radiotherapy, surgical excision, targeted therapy, and biotherapy are often selected for comprehensive intervention. Active treatment can cure more than 30% of cancers, which plays a vital role in delaying cancer progression and prolonging patients' lives. However, we also found that some patients want to seek TCM or integrated Chinese and Western medicine treatment to "enhance effectiveness and reduce toxicity" so as to achieve better therapeutic effects because of their intolerance to the side effects of radiotherapy and chemotherapy, or because of fear of surgery, or because of multiple metastases of advanced cancer.

Cancer belongs to the categories of "cancer disease" and "amassment and accumulation disease" in TCM. In etiology and pathogenesis, zang-fu viscera dysfunction caused by deficiency of vital qi, exogenous pathogenic toxin, emotional internal damage, eating disorders, etc., and internal generation of phlegm, static blood, toxin, etc., caused by poor operation of qi, blood and body fluid, intermingling with each other, lead to cancer with the passage of time. In recent years, Chinese medicinals have played an active role in alleviating adverse reactions of radiotherapy and chemotherapy, relieving cancer-related symptoms, inhibiting tumor growth and metastasis, improving patients' immunity and body function, and patients' quality of life. The clinical value of TCM in treating cancer has been increasingly recognized at home and abroad. This section will focus on TCM's understanding and treatment of lung cancer, liver cancer and gastric cancer.

|| Treatises on malignant tumors

1 Lung cancer

Clinically, we often see some middle-aged and elderly men who smoke with persistent cough and bloody sputum. However, they ignore it until they have apparent chest pain, hemoptysis, and emaciation. Then, they go to the hospital for examination only to find that they have advanced lung cancer. In 2020, more than 2 million people in the world had lung cancer, and nearly 1.8 million people died from it. Lung cancer is also a malignant tumor with the largest number of newly occurring and fatal cases every year in China, which brings a heavy burden to society and patients' families.

Smoking is the most common cause of lung cancer, increasing the risk by an average of 10 times. Besides smoking, air pollution, a poor working environment, and an unhealthy lifestyle are also critical causes of lung cancer.

In clinical manifestations, early lung cancer may not have any symptoms. However, with the progression of the disease, the tumor invades the bronchi, blood vessels, etc., and cough, bloody sputum, and even hemoptysis may occur. Intermediate and advanced lung cancer patients may have apparent symptoms such as emaciation, cough, hemoptysis, shortness of breath, chest pain, fatigue, fever, and hoarseness.

In clinical diagnosis, X-ray chest film, CT, MRI, and other imaging examinations are the most critical means to detect lung cancer and many early lung cancers are found through this. In addition, sputum exfoliated cytology, respiratory endoscopy and lung histopathology are all critical means to diagnose lung cancer.

Clinical treatment mainly includes surgery, drug therapy and radiotherapy. TCM has high clinical value in synergistic effect, alleviating adverse reactions of radiotherapy and chemotherapy, improving immunity and body function, and the quality of life. Therefore, many patients often seek TCM treatment voluntarily.

Lung cancer belongs to the categories of "lung accumulation" and "lung amassment" in TCM. Its etiology is related to insufficiency of congenital endowment, deficiency of vital qi, pathogenic toxin invading the lung, internal accumulation of dampness-phlegm, etc. Its primary pathogenesis is that deficiency of vital qi fails to resist pathogen, dampness-phlegm and pathogenic toxin invades the lung, lung qi fails in dispersing and descending, qi and blood becomes stagnated, and then intermingled phlegm and qi, and static blood contribute to lung cancer with the passage of time.

In clinical treatment, Maimendong Decoction and Aidi Injection, a TCM injection, can be selected. Maimendong Decoction is a famous prescription created by Zhang Zhongjing. It is composed of 6 Chinese medicinals: Maidong (Ophiopogonis Radix), Banxia (Pinelliae Rhizoma), Renshen (Ginseng Radix et Rhizoma), Gancao (Glycyrrhizae Radix et Rhizoma), Jingmi (Oryzae Sativae Semen) and Dazao (Jujubae Fructus). It has the effects of benefiting qi and nourishing yin, and eliminating phlegm and resolving hard mass. Because some symptoms of lung cancer are similar to those of "lung flaccidity" described in the original book, Maimendong Decoction is also used to treat lung cancer patients with manifestations caused by deficiency of both qi and yin, such as cough, shortness of breath, throat discomfort, coughing and spitting turbid phlegm-drool, chest pain, bloody sputum, red tongue, little fur, and feeble and rapid pulse. In use, Biejia (Trionycis Carapax), Banzhilian (Scutellariae Barbatae Herba), Baihuasheshecao (Hedyotis Diffusae Herba), and other Chinese medicinals with anti-cancer and mass-dissipating effects can be added to enhance the curative effects.

Aidi Injection is a kind of Chinese medicinal injection with an anti-cancer effect, which is composed of 4 Chinese medicinals: Renshen (Ginseng Radix et Rhizoma), Huangqi (Astragali Radix), Ciwujia (Acanthopanacis Senticosi Radix et Rhizoma seu Caulis) and Banmao (Mylabris). It has the effects of clearing heat and removing toxicity, and eliminating blood stasis and resolving hard mass. Aidi Injection can be used for postoperative consolidation treatment of primary liver cancer, lung cancer, nasopharyngeal carcinoma, and other tumors. Clinically, it is often used in combination with chemotherapy medicines, which can play a role in enhancing efficacy and attenuating toxicity. A systematic review of 54 clinical trials involving 4,053 patients with non-small cell lung cancer found that Aidi Injection combined with Western medicine chemotherapy significantly improved clinical remission rate and disease control rate, reduced bone marrow suppression, neutropenia, thrombocytopenia, anemia, gastrointestinal reaction and improved liver function. Modern pharmacological studies have found that Aidi Injection can inhibit solid tumors, enhance human immunity and body function, alleviate bone marrow suppression caused by chemotherapy, and maintain the normal levels of white blood cells and platelets.

References

XIAO Z, JIANG Y, WANG C Q, et al. Clinical efficacy and safety of aidi injection combination with vinorelbine and cisplatin for advanced non-small-cell lung carcinoma: a systematic review and meta-analysis of 54 randomized controlled trials[J]. Pharmacol Res, 2020, 153: e104637.

2 Liver cancer

Binge drinking? Smoking? Always eating moldy food? Hepatitis without active treatment? If these behaviors occur, liver cancer may soon find you. In 2020, the number of new cases of liver cancer exceeded 4.5 million in China, accounting for more than 20% of the global total, and the number of deaths exceeded 3 million, accounting for more than 30% of the global total. In addition, the incidence is about 3 times higher in men that in women.

In etiology, viral hepatitis caused by hepatitis B virus infection is the leading cause of liver cancer in China. Frequent consumption of aflatoxin-contaminated food, alcoholism and other causes of liver fibrosis and cirrhosis, and long-term exposure to toxic chemicals are critical causes of liver cancer.

In clinical manifestations, the onset of liver cancer is insidious, with no obvious symptoms in the early stage. When the symptoms are apparent, it is often in the middle or late stage. Middle and advanced liver cancer often presents persistent distending or dull pain in the liver area, progressive enlargement of the liver with hard texture, jaundice, emaciation, poor appetite, and other systemic symptoms.

In clinical diagnosis, it can be definitely diagnosed by histopathological examination of the liver. Liver cancer markers such as alpha-fetoprotein are specific markers for the diagnosis of liver cancer. Ultrasound, enhanced CT, and MRI also play a vital role in the early diagnosis and disease evaluation of liver cancer.

Clinical treatment includes surgery, liver transplantation, radiofrequency ablation, microwave ablation, and targeted therapy, etc. Many patients often seek the help of TCM to obtain a better curative effect.

Liver cancer belongs to the categories of "concretions and conglomerations", "liver amassment" and "tympanites" in TCM. In etiology, it is related to deficiency of vital qi, deficiency of zang-fu viscera, stagnation of seven emotions, invasion of pathogenic toxin, and so on. In pathogenesis, the disorder of yin and yang of zang-fu viscera, poor transportation of qi, blood and fluid, and dysfunction of liver in controlling free flow of qi lead to intermingled phlegm and qi and static blood, and liver cancer occurs with the passage of time.

In clinical treatment, the classic prescription Biejiajian Pill and Kanglaite Injection, a TCM injection, can be selected. Biejiajian Pill comes from *Synopsis of Golden Chamber* written by Zhang Zhongjing. It is composed of 23 Chinese medicinals: Biejia (Trionycis Carapax), Shegan (Belamcandae Rhizoma), Huangqin (Scutellariae Radix), Chaihu (Bupleuri Radix), Shufu (*Armadillidium vulgare*), Ganjiang (Zingiberis Rhizoma), Dahuang (Rhei Radix et Rhizoma), Shaoyao (Paeoniae Radix Alba seu Rubra), Guizhi (Cinnamomi Ramulus), Tinglizi (Descurainiae seu Lepidii Semen), Shiwei (Pyrrosiae Folium), Houpo (Magnoliae Officinalis Cortex), Mudanpi (Moutan Cortex), Qumai (Dianthi Herba), Lingxiaohua (Campsis Flos), Banxia (Pinelliae Rhizoma), Renshen (Ginseng Radix et Rhizoma), Qianglang (*Catharsius molossus*), Tubiechong (Eupolyphaga Steleophaga), Fengfang (Vespae Nidus), Ejiao (Colla Corii Asini), Xiaoshi (Nitre) and Taoren (Persicae Semen). They have the effects of promoting blood circulation to remove blood stasis, softening and resolving hard mass, which is suitable for advanced liver cancer with hard liver texture, uneven surface, multiple nodules, etc. In using, some Chinese medicinals with anti-cancer and mass-resolving effects can be appropriately added, such as Banzhilian (Scutellariae Barbatae Herba) and Baihuasheshecao (Hedyotis Diffusae Herba). Biejiajian Pill has been developed into Chinese patent medicine, and it is a black-brown water-honeyed pill. The dosage and administration method is 3 g orally each time, and 3 times daily.

Kanglaite Injection is extracted from Yiyiren (Coicis Semen). Yiyiren (Coicis Semen) is the dry and mature seed of Gramineae plant *Coix lacryma-jobi* L. var. *ma-yuen* (Roman.) Stapf, which is sweet, tasteless, and slightly cold. It belongs to the spleen, stomach and lung meridians. It has the effects of promoting diuresis, invigorating the spleen, removing bi, clearing heat, and expelling pus. Kanglaite Injection has the effects of invigorating qi and nourishing yin and eliminating concretions and resolving hard mass, and is suitable for patients with primary liver cancer and non-small cell lung cancer, which belongs to deficiency of both qi and yin according to TCM syndrome differentiation. Modern pharmacological studies have found that it can significantly enhance immunity, inhibit the growth of tumor cells, and denaturate tumor cells. Kanglaite Injection is administered by slow intravenous drip, once daily, 200 ml once a day for a course of three weeks.

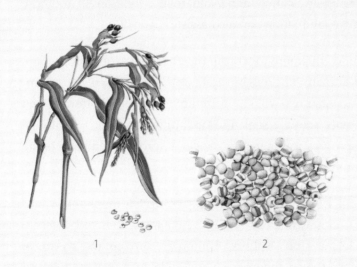

Yiyiren
1. Source plant;
2. decoction pieces.

3 Gastric cancer

Clinically, patients with chronic atrophic gastritis, gastric ulcer, gastric polyps, and other diseases fail to be actively treated and often develop into gastric cancer, bringing tragedy to individuals and their families.

In 2020, the number of new cases of gastric cancer in China was about 479,000, accounting for 10.5% of the total number of new cases of cancer in China, and the number of death cases was about 374,000, accounting for 12.4% of the total number of cancer deaths. Globally, 43.9% of the new cases of gastric cancer and 48.6% of fatal cases of gastric cancer occurred in China.

In etiology, *Helicobacter pylori* infection, chronic atrophic gastritis, intestinal metaplasia, smoking, and heredity are high-risk factors for gastric cancer. Under the comprehensive action of multiple pathogenic factors, "inflammation-cancer transformation" appears, which eventually leads to the occurrence of gastric cancer.

In clinical manifestations, 80% of patients with early gastric cancer have no symptoms, and some may have indigestion. As the disease progresses, many patients may have symptoms such as emaciation, upper abdominal pain, anemia, anorexia, and melena.

In clinical diagnosis, gastroscopy combined with tissue biopsy is the most reliable method to diagnose gastric cancer and evaluate its condition. In addition, tumor markers and imaging examination can also assist diagnosis.

In clinical diagnosis and treatment, according to the condition, endoscopic treatment, surgical resection, chemotherapy, and so on can be taken. However, due to severe adverse reactions and intolerance to radiotherapy and chemotherapy, some patients actively seek TCM treatment to improve clinical discomfort, and delay the progression of gastric cancer, improve the quality of life and prolong the survival time.

In TCM, gastric cancer belongs to the categories of "stomachache" and "dysphagia". In etiology, it is closely related to deficiency of the spleen and stomach, improper diet, insect toxin invasion, emotional internal damage and so on. In pathogenesis, deficiency of the spleen and stomach and imbalance of ascending and descending of qi movement, with phlegm-turbidity, insect toxin, static blood, etc. flowing in the stomach-fu and intermingling with each other, lead to gastric cancer.

In clinical treatment, the classic prescription Banxia Xiexin Decoction and Chinese medicinal injection Cinobufagin Injection are often used. Banxia Xiexin Decoction comes from the *Treatise on Cold Pathogenic Diseases* written by Zhang Zhongjing, a medical sage. It is composed of 7 Chinese medicinals, namely Banxia (Pinelliae Rhizoma), Huanglian (Coptidis Rhizoma), Huangqin (Scutellariae Radix), Renshen (Ginseng Radix et Rhizoma), Ganjiang (Zingiberis Rhizoma), Dazao (Jujubae Fructus) and Gancao (Glycyrrhizae Radix et Rhizoma). It has the effects of mildly regulating cold and heat, dispersing pi and resolving hard mass, and is known as "the first prescription of gastrointestinal diseases". Banxia Xiexin Decoction has a certain effect in treating precancerous lesions of gastric cancer, regulating the microenvironment of gastric cancer, inhibiting tumor growth and relieving stomachache, bloating, acid regurgitation, anorexia, and indigestion. In clinical application, Chinese medicinals with an anti-cancer effect, such as Banzhilian (Scutellariae Barbatae Herba), Baihuasheshecao (Hedyotis Diffusae Herba), Shancigu (Cremastrae seu Pleiones Pseudobulbus), Guijianyu (Euonymi Ramulus), etc., can be combined as appropriate.

Cinobufagin Injection is a kind of Chinese medicinal injection with anti-cancer effect, which is processed from the whole dried skin of *Bufo bufo gargarizans* Cantor in the shade. Toad skin has the effects of clearing heat and removing toxicity, inducing diuresis to alleviate edema. It can be used for carbuncle and deep-rooted carbuncle, scrofula, tumor, and other diseases. A meta-analysis of 27 clinical trials involving 1,939 cases of advanced gastric cancer showed that, compared with chemotherapy alone, the combination of cinobufagin not only significantly improved overall remission rate and disease control rate, but also alleviated adverse reactions such as nausea and vomiting, diarrhea, leukopenia and peripheral neurotoxicity caused by chemotherapy. Modern pharmacological studies have found that cinobufagin can inhibit tumor cell proliferation, induce tumor cell apoptosis and inhibit tumor neovascularization.

References

SUN H, WANG W, BAI M, et al. Cinobufotalin as an effective adjuvant therapy for advanced gastric cancer: a meta-analysis of randomized controlled trials[J]. Onco Targets Ther, 2019, 12: 3139-3160.

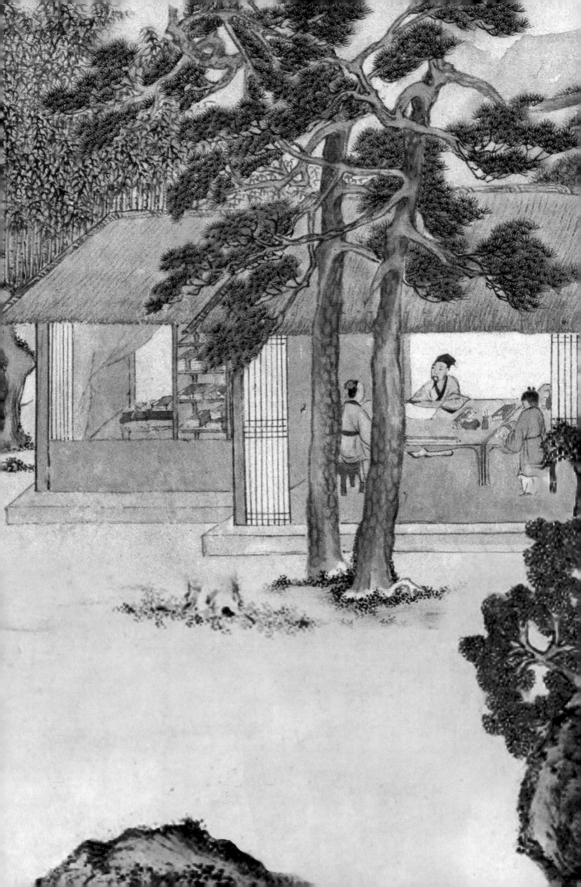

Chapter 3

The Prospect of Clinical Diagnosis and

Treatment of TCM

President Xi Jinping emphasizes that "it is necessary to follow the development law of TCM, and inherit the essence, with cultural inheritance and innovation". There are many academic schools and viewpoints in TCM, but not all are the "essence". However, the TCM classic book *Treatise on Cold Pathogenic Diseases* and the effective prescriptions handed down by later famous Chinese medicine doctors must be the "essence" of TCM. Therefore, we often refer to the classic prescriptions in the *Treatise on Cold Pathogenic Diseases* by Zhang Zhongjing. The prescriptions are widely circulated and used in later generations as classic prescriptions. For example, we are familiar with Xiaochaihu Decoction/Granule for treating fever, Maxing Shigan Decoction/Tablet for treating acute bronchitis and pneumonia, Xiaoyao Pill/Granule for treating female chest pain and breast nodules, Liuwei Dihuang Pill and Shenqi Pill for treating kidney deficiency and low back pain, etc. Compared with the self-made prescriptions commonly used in the clinic, the classic prescriptions are superior in both efficacy and safety. Many Chinese patent medicines and TCM injections used in modern clinics come from classic prescriptions.

"Innovation" means that under the guidance of TCM theory, we apply Chinese medicinals, acupuncture, massage, and other TCM treatment methods to solve current clinical medical problems. Many people may think that Western medicine is so powerful, is there still be a clinical problem that cannot be solved? In fact, in clinical practice, we will encounter many diseases that Western medicine can't help. First of all, corona virus disease 2019 (COVID-19) is a vivid example. TCM and integration of Chinese and Western medicine play a vital role during the treatment (Pharmacol Res 2020). In addition, for various viral infectious diseases, including influenza A, SARS, etc., the antiviral and symptomatic support treatment of Western medicine is not effective. Second, in the early stage of many diseases, including prehypertension, prediabetes (impaired glucose tolerance), precancerous lesions, pulmonary nodules (<8 mm), and other diseases, Western medicine is still lack of effective treatment methods. Third, for the diseases, including rheumatic immune system diseases, immunosuppressants and hormones are routinely used. However, the effects are limited with toxic side effects and patients' intolerance. Fourth, in terms of functional diseases, including autonomic nerve dysfunction, cardiac neurosis, and even some diseases from which patients suffer a lot, but no significant abnormality is found during examination, TCM has a confirmed efficacy.

Fortunately, in recent years, the clinical advantages of TCM have been gradually recognized internationally. High-quality clinical evidences have been gradually obtained China in various fields, such as Tianqi Jiangtang Capsule for the treatment of impaired glucose tolerance; acupuncture for the treatment of mixed urinary incontinence, female stress urinary incontinence, chronic refractory constipation, chronic prostatitis/chronic pelvic floor pain syndrome, and benign prostatic hyperplasia; Maren Pill for the treatment of constipation; Chinese medicinals for the treatment of ulcerative colitis; Tai Chi for the treatment of rheumatoid arthritis. In addition, for other diseases, including dizziness, insomnia, anxiety, etc., although high-quality evidence has not been obtained, good curative effect has been achieved in daily clinical work in hospitals, which is also worthy of attention.